Vaccine Intervention Against Virus-induced Tumours

LEUKAEMIA AND LYMPHOMA RESEARCH

Vaccine Intervention against Virus-induced Tumours

Edited by

J. M. Goldman
Consultant Physician
Royal Postgraduate Medical School
Hammersmith Hospital
London W12 0HS, UK

and

M. A. Epstein
Professor of Pathology
University of Bristol Medical School
Bristol BS8 1TD, UK

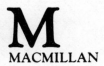

MACMILLAN

First published 1986

Published in Great Britain by
THE MACMILLAN PRESS LTD
Houndmills, Basingstoke, Hampshire RG21 2XS
and London
Companies and representatives
throughout the world

Distributed in North America by
SHERIDAN HOUSE PUBLISHERS
145 Palisade Street, Dobbs Ferry, NY 10522

Printed in Great Britain by
Camelot Press Ltd,
Southampton

British Library Cataloguing in Publication Data
Vaccine intervention against virus-induced
tumours.—(Leukaemia and lymphoma research)
1. Viral carcinogenesis   2. Tumors—
Preventive inoculation
I. Goldman, John M.   II. Epstein, M. A.   III. Series
614.5'999   RC268.57
ISBN 0-333-39830-0

Contents

The Contributors

E. Beth-Giraldo
Division of Viral Oncology
Pascale Institute
80131 Naples
Italy

P. M. Biggs
Houghton Poultry Research Station
Houghton, Huntingdon
Cambs PE17 2DA
UK

B. S. Blumberg
Institute for Cancer Research
7701 Burholme Avenue, Fox Chase
Philadelphia, PA 19111
USA

D. P. Bolognesi
Building 37, Rm 6A09
NIH, National Cancer Institute
Bethesda, Maryland 20205
USA

M. A. Epstein
Department of Pathology
University of Bristol Medical School
Bristol BS8 1TD
UK

P. J. Fischinger
Building 37, Rm 6A09
NIH, National Cancer Institute
Bethesda, Maryland 20205
USA

R. C. Gallo
Building 37, Rm 6A09
NIH, National Cancer Institute
Bethesda, Maryland 20205
USA

G. Giraldo
Division of Viral Oncology
Pascale Institute
80131 Naples
Italy

H. zur Hausen
Cancer Research Centre
Im Neuenheimer Feld 280
D-6900 Heidelberg 1
West Germany

L. J. N. Ross
Houghton Poultry Research Station
Houghton, Huntingdon
Cambs PE17 2DA
UK

A. J. Zuckerman
Department of Medical Microbiology
London School of Hygiene and Tropical Medicine
Keppel Street
London WC1E 7HT

Preface

This volume is the third in the series entitled *Leukaemia and Lymphoma Research,* which was initiated in 1984. The Annual Guest Lecture, around which the volume was constructed, was delivered by Professor M. A. Epstein, and reviewed his work culminating in the development of a vaccine that can prevent virus-induced lymphomas in tamarin monkeys. Thus he and the other contributors to this volume describe, in varying degrees of detail, the progress of efforts to prevent selected malignant diseases in man and animals by use of purpose-made vaccines.

To the newcomer, the surprise might be not so much that viruses can cause (or be co-factors in causing) leukaemias, lymphomas and solid tumours in man, but that it took so long for the general principle to be acknowledged by the scientific community. The history is long enough. Viruses, of course, are a comparatively recent concept, but filterable agents (ill-defined agents smaller than the smallest known bacteria that could traverse asbestos filter pads or unglazed porcelain filter candles) were known since the end of the last century. In 1908 Ellermann and Bang in Copenhagen succeeded in transmitting erythromyeloblastic leukaemia in chickens by transfer of filterable material from affected birds; three years later, Peyton Rous at the Rockefeller Institute in New York, transmitted the first solid tumour (a sarcoma) from diseased chickens to normal recipients. (He received a Nobel prize for this work only in 1965.)

There then followed a long interval during which there were no further reports of leukaemia or solid tumours transmitted by filterable agents. In the early 1930s, however, Richard Shope in New Jersey reported the transmission of rabbit fibroma by filtrates, and subsequently transmission of rabbit papillomas. In 1936 John Bittner at Bar Harbor reported that an agent capable of causing mouse mammary carcinoma could be transmitted through the milk of nursing female mice. Two years later Baldwin Lucké in Philadelphia provided evidence that a kidney carcinoma of frogs was caused by a transmissible virus.

In the 1950s much evidence accumulated linking various RNA-containing viruses with tumours and leukaemias in rodents. Ludwig Gross reported in 1951 that filtrates from 'infected' animals could transmit leukaemia in mice, and in

1957 Stewart and Eddy at the National Cancer Institute defined an agent (a polyoma virus) capable of causing parotid tumours in new-born mice. In 1957, Charlotte Friend at the Sloan Kettering Institute in New York, isolated a filterable agent that could induce an erythroblastosis-like syndrome in weanling mice. In 1960 Eddy and Girardi separately reported that a simian virus (SV40) could cause sarcomas in new-born hamsters. In 1962 John Trentin showed that an adenovirus could also induce sarcomas in hamsters. In 1964 William Jarrett reported the transmission by a virus of leukaemia/lymphoma in cats. This is a very incomplete catalogue of the landmarks of the first fifty-odd years of viral oncology, but it serves to illustrate how spasmodic was the progress. Initially the concept that viruses could cause malignant disease was discounted by almost all; subsequently many accepted that viruses could, in isolated or experimental situations, cause tumours in animals, but they believed that the examples were irrelevant to man.

Much has now changed over the last 20 years. Perhaps the new era dawned with the demonstration in 1964 of a new herpes-like virus (now named EBV) associated with characteristic lymphoma described originally by Denis Burkitt in East African children. Though rigorous proof that this agent causes Burkitt's lymphoma is not yet available, the circumstantial evidence in favour is compelling. In the 1970s, one of the causative agents of infectious hepatitis (the hepatitis B virus) was identified and this now seems to be a major co-factor in the aetiology of hepatocarcinoma in many parts of the world, perhaps less so in Europe and North America. One of the later pieces of the jigsaw is the recognition of a distinctive RNA virus, termed ATV or HTLV-1, as a probable cause of adult T-cell leukaemia lymphoma in Japan and the Caribbean. Though one must immediately concede that the evidence linking viruses with the bulk of common human tumours is weak or non-existent, it is now clear nonetheless that some tumours would almost certainly not have occurred if a specific co-factor, in this case the virus, were deleted from the environment or at least eradicated from the body.

This then is the background for attempts to immunise susceptible humans against the potential leukaemogenic or carcinogenic effects of different viruses. To my knowledge this is the first attempt to assemble under one cover details of the various vaccinal approaches to the prevention of human and animal tumors. I hope the reader will find this volume informative and to some extent also entertaining. I hope it points the way to important therapeutic advances in the future.

I thank all the authors for their contributions. They were all delivered before or very soon after the specified date. Editors are always very grateful when the targets are achieved by all.

London, April 1986 J. M. G.
M. A. E.

The Leukaemia Research Fund

The Leukaemia Research Fund is the only national charitable foundation in Britain devoting all its resources to research and patient care in leukaemia and the related blood diseases. Founded in 1960, it is the third largest cancer organisation in Britain and is a member of the United Kingdom Co-ordinating Committee on Cancer Research. The Fund is advised by a distinguished Medical and Scientific Advisory Panel.

The Fund finances an expanding programme of research and has recently set up the Leukaemia Research Fund Centre at the Institute of Cancer Research in London for the study of the molecular and cellular biology of human leukaemia. It has also introduced a large-scale progressive aetiology study in Britain with particular emphasis on the biology of the diseases, and has funded pioneering work in Britain on bone-marrow transplantation. In addition, the Fund is involved in the clinical support of patients and provides a full information service. Its academic work, including international symposia, workshops and lectures, is complemented by an active policy of world-wide collaboration. The Leukaemia Research Fund Annual Guest Lecture is delivered by a scientist or doctor who has made a major contribution to knowledge of leukaemia and lymphomas.

Hepatitis B Virus and Primary Cancer of the Liver

Introduction

In this introductory chapter the use of vaccines to intervene against virus-induced tumours will be discussed, the hepatitis B virus (HBV) and its causative role in primary hepatocellular carcinoma (PHC) being used as an example.

The vaccine which is currently in use will be discussed first. There will follow a summary of the evidence supporting the hypothesis that HBV is the cause of PHC. (This topic will be discussed in greater detail in Chapter 4 in this volume.) The consequence of accepting this hypothesis will then be considered. There are unusual features of the HBV–PHC relation which are not explained by current viral cancer models. A model introduced by London and Blumberg[1,2] to explain these relations will be presented. The model is of heuristic value, in that it suggests interesting experiments and novel approaches to diagnosis and therapy which may have application to other virus-caused cancers. A broad description of the public health and clinical programmes in progress and planned will then be given.

Each time a medical solution is introduced, it raises other problems, many of which were not anticipated. The prevention of HBV infection is no exception. As an example of such a problem, the possible role of HBV in the determination of the sex of the offspring of infected parents and how this may be affected by vaccination programmes will be briefly reviewed. This interesting biological and medical phenomenon may also occur with other viruses.

Vaccines

Evidence has been accumulating since the early 1970s[3,4] supporting the hypothesis that persistent infection with HBV is required for the development of the disease: that is, that HBV is a necessary cause of PHC. There is now substantial support for this hypothesis. Massive public health programmes are in place or planned, to prevent infection with HBV and thereby, presumably, prevent primary cancer of the liver as well as acute and chronic liver disease due to HBV, which are major causes of morbidity and mortality in areas of the world where the largest populations reside, including sub-Saharan Africa, Asia and Oceania. PHC is probably the major cause, or one of the major causes, of death from cancer in men in the world, and these programmes, therefore, should have a major impact on cancer prevention comparable to the expected effects of cessation of cigarette smoking on cancer of the lung.

Shortly after the discovery of what subsequently became designated as hepatitis B virus, it was recognised that large amounts of the viral surface antigen (HBsAg) were present in the blood of carriers of HBV in separate particles which apparently contained no viral nucleic acid, which did not replicate and which were not infectious. In 1969 Blumberg and Millman introduced a novel vaccine prepared from these particles[5]. The surface antigen particles of HBV were separated from the blood of carriers by centrifugation and other means. They were then treated in a variety of ways to inactivate any remaining hepatitis B virus, or any other viruses which may exist in the blood, and the resulting material was incorporated in the vaccine preparation. In 1971 arrangements were made with the Merck Company to develop and manufacture the vaccine, and they and other companies in several parts of the world are now producing sufficient quantities to supply the needs of the public health programmes and for other uses.

A series of field trials of the vaccine – in particular, that of Szmuness and his colleagues[6] in 1980 – demonstrated that the vaccine was highly effective and offered protection in more than 90% of those vaccinated; it was, within the limits of the study, entirely safe. Since the initial field trials, additional observations have been made and, to date, no deleterious side-effects of the vaccine have been found. It is possible that more than 2 million doses of the vaccine prepared from human blood have now been used; hence, on the basis of available information, this appears to be one of the safest vaccines ever introduced. In particular, it has been shown that the isolation and purification process inactivates HTLV-III, the retrovirus thought to be the cause of acquired immune deficiency syndrome (AIDS)[7-9].

Hepatitis vaccines have recently been prepared by recombinant DNA methods. The gene for the surface antigen, including the pre-S region of the genome adjacent to it, has been cloned in yeast and other organisms. Large quantities of surface antigen are produced by this process. The surface antigen is separated from the yeast and its products are purified and used as the vaccine. Several investigators have shown that the resultant material is antigenic and produces significant amounts of anti-HBs in humans. Protection studies are now in progress to determine whether the recombinant vaccine is as effective and safe as the currently used product produced from human blood. If the new vaccine is also as safe as the present vaccine (which may take several years to determine), then, if the cost is less, it may replace the 'natural' product. Other forms of vaccines have also been conceived and prepared, and these will be discussed elsewhere in this volume.

A Summary of the Evidence that Hepatitis B Virus is a Necessary Cause of Primary Hepatocellular Carcinoma

There is now a substantial body of evidence to support the hypothesis that persistent infection with HBV is required for the development of most cases of PHC. These data have been reviewed in many articles (see Blumberg and London[2], where references to original studies may be found).

When the most sensitive methods are used, infection with HBV is found in about 90% or more of cases of PHC; that is, the attributable risk is extremely high. An interesting feature of these observations is that the amount of surface antigen detectable in the peripheral blood decreases as the cancer proceeds; the more cancer cells present in the host, the less virus is found in the peripheral blood. HBV can be identified in the liver cells in a very high percentage of the PHC cases. From the time of the earliest observations, it was noted that the surface antigen, whole virus and core antigen are much more common in the liver cells which are not 'transformed' (i.e. do not have the appearance of a cancer cell) than in the cells which are.

The HBV DNA is integrated into the DNA of the host liver cells in patients with cancer. Integration is found both in the cells in which 'malignant transformation' has occurred and in cells without evidence of cancer. Some investigators have reported that integration of HBV DNA into host DNA is also seen in individuals who do not have cancer: that is, patients with chronic liver disease or asymptomatic persons who have been carriers of HBV for a long time. Hence, integration *per se* is not a sufficient explanation of cancer causation.

HBV DNA does not include an oncogene. In most cases there are multiple integrated copies of the HBV genome in the liver cells of patients with cancer. In any given tumour the site(s) of integration in each cell are the same (i.e. the integration appears to be clonal), but there is no uniform site of integration when different tumours are compared. There is at present no evidence for integration related to an oncogene site in the host and oncogene theory is not required to explain the pathogenesis of PHC. However, sufficient studies have not been completed to reveal a possibly more complex relation of HBV integration to an oncogene, or to other genes.

A series of convincing epidemiological studies, some of them discussed elsewhere in this volume, have added substantially to the evidence that HBV is a necessary cause of PHC. Beasley and his co-workers in Taiwan[10] found in a prospective study that asymptomatic carriers of HBV had a much higher risk of developing PHC than controls selected from the same population; the relative risk was more than 200:1. Hence, HBV carriers in this environment and probably in others are one of the highest risk groups for any of the common cancers. By comparison, the relative risk for cancer of the lung among cigarette smokers is about 30:1. It has also been shown that among patients with chronic liver disease (CLD) it is those with CLD due to HBV that are at highest risk of developing PHC, but the risk is not greatly increased in patients with CLD due to other causes. None of these data excludes the possibility that there may be other necessary 'causes' of PHC. For example, toxins such as aflatoxin may interact with the liver and/or HBV to accelerate the development of a cancer, and studies of this process are planned and in progress.

Progression from HBV to Chronic Liver Disease and Primary Hepatocellular Carcinoma

In regions of the world where HBV and PHC are common, infection can occur very early in life, before birth or at the time of birth. However, even though infection may occur early, HBsAg and HBV are not persistent in the blood until 2–3 months of age. This gap is providential, since it allows for the effective vaccination of the offspring of carrier mothers very soon after birth. In parts of Asia maternal transmission is particularly common. Nishioka has estimated that it is responsible for about 40% or more of all carriers in Japan[4]. In Africa maternal transmission appears to be less common, but infection usually occurs in early childhood (say the first 5 years) as a consequence of exposure to carriers in the family and later to other members of the extended community[11]. Children, when exposed to infection at a young age, are more likely to become carriers than if they are exposed at a later age, when they are more likely to develop anti-HBs. Hence, protection against childhood infection is particularly important in the prevention of the carrier state.

Carriers may remain asymptomatic for many years. However, in most carriers of HBV the invasion of liver cells by HBV and cell death may be occurring at a slow rate. This destruction can increase with time, and liver cell death can lead to regeneration, scarring and the pathological and clinical picture of chronic liver disease. Some individuals who survive the effects of chronic liver disease will proceed to develop primary hepatocellular carcinoma. This is usually a disease of short duration, even with treatment, and death intervenes within a few months or years of diagnosis. Not every infected person becomes a carrier, and not every carrier develops chronic liver disease and/or goes on to develop PHC. Hence, other factors (for example, aflatoxin) may intervene at these 'decision' points to determine the fate of an individual carrier.

The R–S Developmental Model for HBV–PHC Relation

London and Blumberg have devised a cellular model to account for the observed epidemiological, clinical, biological and molecular features of the HBV–PHC relationship[1]. This model, which has some unusual features, is of heuristic value in that it suggests novel experiments and, possibly, treatments. It may also serve as a guide to the interpretation of other virus–cancer relations discussed elsewhere in this volume.

The model postulates the existence of two types of liver cells, 'R' and 'S', with respect to infection with HBV. The R cell is an undifferentiated or less differentiated hepatocyte capable of division, common in fetal life, less common in the newborn and rare in the adult. In the fetus it provides for the growth of the liver, and in the adult the occasional R cells provide the source of dividing cells required for the replacement of liver cells lost through damage or disease. Normally, when R cells divide, they form one R and one S cell. If differentiation is perturbed, one R cell could yield two S cells, which would remove that lineage as source for further cell replacement, or a defect in differentiation could yield two R cells, two cells capable of further division.

The S cells are differentiated hepatocytes which compose most of the parenchymal cells of adult liver. They have limited ability to divide but can support replication of HBV. When they do divide, they form only other differentiated S cells. Integration of HBV DNA into S-cell DNA may occur during chronic infection. Viral replication in the S cells eventually leads to the death of many infected S cells, either through a direct effect on the cell or, more likely, as a consequence of the host response to the infected cell. When R cells are infected, complete replication of the virus does not occur, but integration of HBV DNA into R-cell DNA may occur. Hence, the R cells are not destroyed by the replicating virus and are at a selective advantage. (Thus, 'S' signifies susceptible to and R-resistant to replicative infection with HBV.)

The death of S cells stimulates the division of R cells. At some point a 'second event' may occur allowing of the formation of favoured clones of R cells. The development of such a clone may be the result of a particular site (or sites) of HBV DNA integration, or may be the consequence of an environmental or other carcinogen. For example, the HBV DNA integration could occur in a manner to stimulate growth factor production or be proximate to an oncogene. (There is no experimental confirmation of such an integration.) The 'second event' may initiate an irreversible or difficult-to-reverse defect in differentiation in which proliferation of R cells produces only other R cells. This finally results in a tumour mass perceptible to the patient which produces symptoms, local spread, metastasis and death.

This model explains the unusual features of PHC seen at a clinical, population, cellular and molecular level. Time is a major element in the model. The early-childhood infection and its chronicity give time for the infection of S cells, the replication of HBV within them and their subsequent death, leading to liver scarring, regeneration and dysfunction. This could explain the pathogenesis of chronic liver disease and post-hepatic cirrhosis. This also explains the observation that virions of HBV are not seen in cancer cells, which in the model are derived from R cells. HBV proteins and virions are seen in the non-cancer cells, which are the equivalent of the S cells of the model. Cellular division of R cells gives increased opportunity for the 'second event' to occur some time after infection. The favoured clone, which can be formed by the second event, results in R cells which produce only other R cells. After this second event occurs, a stage of the disease ensues which is difficult to slow down, stop or reverse. Hence, remedial action would be best undertaken before the second event.

As time passes during the course of HBV-induced chronic liver disease, there are fewer S cells in the liver. These are replaced by R cells, not vulnerable to death from HBV infection. This explains the decreased amount of HBsAg, HBeAg (an indicator of viral replication) and whole virus present in the peripheral blood as the disease progresses. In the later stages of the disease, when very few S cells remain, much of the liver function available to the host would be supplied by the R cells.

The model may also explain why HBV is not seen during the first few months after birth, even if infection occurs during fetal life. In the fetus and newborn, R cells, in which replication cannot occur, will predominate. Hence, if the fetus or newborn is infected, only a few S cells would be available in which replication occurs, but at such a low level that it is not detectable in the peripheral blood. As the liver matures, more S cells are formed (by division of the R cells), and at about 2-3 months a sufficient number of S cells are present to allow of replication at a level which produces quantities of virus which are detectable in the peripheral blood. (For a description of what appears to be a similar process in ducks infected with duck hepatitis B virus, see Reference 12.) The concurrent presence of R cells, although fewer in number than at or before birth, provides a ready source for recruitment of additional S cells (to replace those killed by viral replication) which can sustain a chronic infection; hence, young people have a propensity for chronic infection.

This model may have application to other virus–cancer relations in which phenomena similar to the HBV–PHC relation are found. Several of these can be mentioned here.

1. The virus is associated both with cancer (PHC) and with other non-malignant diseases (acute hepatitis, post-hepatic cirrhosis, persistent liver disease and, possibly, periarteritis nodosa).

2. There is a very long 'latent' period for the development of the cancer. The initial infection may occur in childhood but the cancer is not perceived until adulthood.

3. Small numbers of cancer cells and, in some cases, products of these cells may be found long before there is a clinical appreciation of the disease. In PHC, α-fetoprotein can be detected in the peripheral blood many years before a perceptible tumour is detected, and tissue and serum ferritins are also early predictors of impending cancer.

4. There are two classes of cells in respect to replicative infection. In one, integration may occur but replication does not. In the other, integration may or may not occur, but replication and subsequently death of the cell does. (In the model these are, respectively, the R and S cells.) The virus may act in the pathogenesis of PHC both by killing the S cells and, in the R cells, when integration occurs, by leading to the selection of a clone which acquires cancer-like properties.

These findings suggest alternatives to the usual forms of cancer therapy. Individuals at high risk — that is, persistent carriers of HBV — can be identified at a very early age. The model suggests that the death of the S cells (fully differentiated cells) stimulates the division of the R cells (less differentiated cells), which in due course leads to the 'second event' and cancer. Hence, prevention can be directed towards *preventing* the death of S cells rather than attempting to kill cancer or pre-cancer cells. How can this be done? Several methods suggest themselves, and research is currently in progress to investigate these possibilities. They include a search for agents which can stop or decrease replication of the virus, and several promising candidates have been found. In the early stages of infection — say in the first few years of the carrier state — integration may not occur or may be only a rare event. An antivirotic may be effective at this period, since it would not have to remove the viral DNA from the host liver cell genome in order to be effective.

There are probably specific surface sites through which HBV enters the liver cells. Recent studies on the polymerised serum albumin binding site of the virus suggest that this may be related to cell wall attachment and entry. However, there is no direct evidence for this, and other sites may be involved. If these can be identified, then steps to deny entry of the virus may be possible. Modifying the cell milieu to decrease the replication of virus may also be feasible. For example, a variety of studies indicate that lowered cellular and storage iron levels may inhibit viral replication.

These procedures may eliminate the virus from the carrier — in particular, shortly after the carrier state has been initiated. If this is not possible, they may slow down the process of viral replication, cell invasion and destruction to such a degree that the pathogenic process will be slowed down and the carrier may survive to a normal life-span. We have termed this 'prevention by delay'.

Primary and Secondary Prevention

Major programmes for primary prevention — that is, prevention of initial infection by the virus — are now in progress, and even larger regional and national programmes are planned. They depend primarily on the vaccination of newborns and infants. In areas of low and intermediate endemicity of carriers (for example, in Japan, where the frequency of carriers is about 1–3%), pregnant women are screened to identify carriers. The carriers are then tested to determine those who also are HBeAg(+) (that is, highly infectious), and hyperimmune gammaglobulin is given to the child at birth. A vaccination programme of three injections over a period of 6 months is begun at 3 months of age; this regimen provides a very high degree of protection. Thousands of children have been given prophylactic treatment in this programme.

In Philadelphia a similar project is in progress. There are about 110 000 people of Asian origin in the Delaware Valley (the geographic region in which

Philadelphia is located), and screening studies have shown that the frequency of carriers is about the same as in their homeland (from 5% to about 15%). Pregnant women are being screened, and offspring of all carrier mothers (not just those who are HBeAg(+)) are offered prophylaxis. In this programme many children have been spared the clinical and psychological pain of becoming carriers.

In some areas, such as China or the Gambia in West Africa, where the frequency of carriers is very high (10–15%), it is planned to vaccinate all children irrespective of the carrier state of their mothers. In these communities the sources of infection are numerous and varied, and the offspring of non-carrier mothers are also at high risk.

In some programmes adult vaccination is also planned. For example, in Alaska the authorities are vaccinating all native Americans (that is, Eskimos, Aleuts and Indians), since the hepatitis carrier state is high in this community. In Philadelphia vaccination is being offered to the family and household members of individuals who are found to be carriers. Regional programmes are in progress in several regions of Italy (Lombardy, Tuscany) and other programmes are being planned (Campania). The World Bank is funding the construction of factories in the People's Republic of China for the manufacture of vaccine from the blood of carriers. This will be used in what promises to be the largest programme in the world, the vaccination of the children (and possibly the adults) of China, with a population of over one billion people. There are other programmes planned or in place in South Korea, Taiwan, Singapore and elsewhere.

Some of the regions with the greatest need for hepatitis vaccination are those with the smallest public health budgets: for example, countries of sub-Saharan Africa. We and other workers in the field have recommended an internationally funded programme, similar to that successfully applied to the elimination of smallpox, and the international medical organisations have proposed such programmes.

Many of the national and regional programmes will have special or even unique features. It is to be hoped that each project can be organised to allow scientific study of the public health strategies and provide valuable information for subsequent programmes.

Secondary Prevention

As already noted, hepatitis B carriers are at high risk of developing PHC. Chinese investigators have reported that early tumours, usually not perceptible to the individual, can be detected by the serial measurement of α-fetoprotein (AFP)[13]. Sustained elevations of AFP may indicate the presence of malignant cells; visualisation techniques (such as ultrasound, CAT scan, etc.) can then be used to determine whether a tumour is actually present. Surgery can then be offered to the carriers. Preliminary studies have shown that there is an increased survival rate in those who have a successful removal compared with those who refuse surgery[13].

Additional long-term prospective studies will be required to confirm the early Asian investigations, particularly in America, Africa and Europe, where the factors contributing to pathogenesis may be different. If this procedure does in fact prolong life (rather than apparently doing so because of earlier detection), then detection and monitoring of carriers may become a widely used procedure for the prevention of PHC. The carriers apparently remain at high risk of developing another tumour after the first has been removed, and continual monitoring after surgery may be required.

Hepatitis B Virus, Fertility and Sex Ratio

A study of the history of medicine teaches us that each time a problem is solved it usually generates one or more new ones. When these, in turn, are resolved, they can generate additional questions and problems; hence, although conditions can be improved, they can rarely be made perfect.

In this section a curious biological characteristic of HBV in relation to sex ratio of humans will be discussed to provide an example of a biological problem that might result from widespread vaccination programmes. These findings are not a contraindication to prevention programmes, since the decrease in morbidity and mortality could be enormous if these programmes are successful. However, the observations which have been made on sex ratio and fertility should be considered as the vaccination programmes develop.

Males and females respond somewhat differently to infection with hepatitis B virus. Males are more likely to become carriers and females to develop anti-HBs when infected with HBV. The response of parents to HBV infection also appears to be measurably related to the sex ratio of their offspring. (Sex ratio is defined as the number of male children at birth divided by the number of females ever born multiplied by 100.) In families where either parent is a carrier of HBV (HBsAg(+)) and the mother does not have anti-HBs (designated 'carrier families') the sex ratio of the offspring is greater than in families where the mother has anti-HBs ('antibody families'). The sex ratio is intermediate in the families in which neither parent has evidence of infection. The difference in ratio is due primarily to a deficit of girls; the carrier and antibody families have about the same number of boys, but the antibody families have a greater number of girls[14-18].

In countries with large families the difference in fertility between the carrier and antibody families is nearly one daughter. There is also an overall effect on fertility. The carrier families have smaller overall numbers of children than the antibody families, and this can be accounted for by a deficiency of females.

These studies have now been conducted in four very different communities: (1) Plati, a small town in Greek Macedonia[14]; (2) Kar Kar, an island off the north coast of Papua New Guinea[15]; (3) Matas Na Kahoy, a village on the island of Luzon in the Philippines[16]; and (4) two small Eskimo communities on the east coast of Greenland[17]. The results from each of these are generally in agreement, but they cannot be extrapolated to other populations where HBV carriers occur in high frequency (such as China or Africa) until similar observations are made in these areas.

Would widespread public health vaccination programmes alter this unusual relation between HBV and human sex, and, if so, what effects could be anticipated? It is not known whether the effects on sex ratio of vaccine-induced anti-HBs will be the same as those of naturally occurring antibody. However, if these results are confirmed and the effects are altered by vaccination, then it would be important to be aware of this phenomenon. In some traditional and other societies boys are more valued than girls; an alteration in sex ratio in the community may therefore have sociological, psychological and economic impact.

As noted, even if those sex ratio effects are influenced by vaccination, it is unlikely that they would counterbalance the beneficial effects of vaccination in decreasing the considerable morbidity and mortality which results from acute and chronic infection with HBV.

Conclusions

The aetiological role of HBV in the development of PHC has been substantially supported. A safe and effective vaccine is available and widely used. Public health programmes for the prevention of liver disease and primary hepatocellular carcinoma are now in progress. A model of how HBV 'causes' PHC has been introduced which has some unusual features, including suggestions for new approaches to prevention and treatment. These concepts may be useful in considering other virus–cancer relations, and their prevention and treatment.

Acknowledgements

This work was supported by USPHS grants CA-06551, RR-05539 and CA-06927 from the National Institutes of Health, and by an appropriation from the Commonwealth of Pennsylvania.

References

1. London WT, Blumberg BS (1983) Hepatitis B and related viruses in chronic hepatitis, cirrhosis and hepatocellular carcinoma in man and animals. In: Cohen S, Soloway RD (eds) Chronic active liver disease. Churchill Livingstone, New York, p 147–170
2. Blumberg BS, London WT (1985) Guest Editorial. Hepatitis B virus and the prevention of primary cancer of the liver. Journal of the National Cancer Institute 74: 267–273
3. Blumberg BS, Larouze B, London WT, Werner B, Hesser JE, Millman I, Saimot G, Payet M (1975) The relation of infection with the hepatitis B agent to primary hepatic carcinoma. American Journal of Pathology 81: 669–682

4. Nishioka K, Hirayama T, Sekine T, Okochi K, Mayumi M, Sung J-L, Liu C-H, Lin T-M (1973) Australia antigen and hepatocellular carcinoma. GANN Monograph on Cancer Research 14: 167–175
5. Blumberg BS, Millman I (1972) Patent. Vaccine against viral hepatitis and process. Submitted October 8, 1969. US Patent Office No 3,636,191, 1972
6. Szmuness W, Stevens CE, Harley EJ, Zang EA, Oleszko WR, William DC, Sadovsky R, Morrison JM, Kellner A (1980) Hepatitis B vaccine: Demonstration of efficacy in a controlled clinical trial in a high-risk population in the United States. New England Journal of Medicine 303: 833–841
7. Kessler H, Chase R, Harris A, Jensen D, Levin S (1985) HTLV–III antibodies after hepatitis B vaccination. Lancet 1: 1506–1507
8. Poisz B, Tomar R, Lehr B, Moore J (1984) Hepatitis B vaccine: evidence confirming lack of AIDS transmission. Morbidity and Mortality Weekly Report 33: 685–687
9. Kirschbaum A, Salomon A, Parker E, Abarca V, Contreras L, Chomali M, Dinator R, Escobar L, Fabre V, Gelman M, Gutierrez V, Hazbun M, Murillo V, Opazo A, Riveros T, Samman M (1985) Recommendations for protection against viral hepatitis. Recommendation of the Immunization Practices Advisory Committee (ACIP). Morbidity and Mortality Weekly Report 34: 314–335
10. Beasley RP, Lin C–C, Hwang L–Y, Chien C–S (1981) Hepatocellular carcinoma and hepatitis B virus: A prospective study of 22,707 men in Taiwan. Lancet 2: 1129–1133
11. Marinier E, Barrois V, Larouze B, London WT, Cofer A, Diakhate L, Blumberg BS (1985) Lack of perinatal transmission of hepatitis B virus infection in Senegal, West Africa. Journal of Pediatrics 106: 843–849
12. Urban MK, O'Connell AP, London WT (1985) Sequence of events in natural infection of Pekin duck embryos with duck hepatitis B virus. Journal of Virology 55: 16–22
13. Tang Z, Yang B, Tang C, Yu Y, Lin Z, Weng H (1980) Evaluation of population screening for hepatocellular carcinoma. Chinese Medical Journal 93: 795–799
14. Drew JS, London WT, Lustbader ED, Hesser JE, Blumberg BS (1978) Hepatitis B virus and sex ratio of offspring. Science 201: 687–692
15. Drew J, London WT, Blumberg BS, Serjeantson S (1982) Hepatitis B virus and sex ratio on Kar Kar Island. Human Biology 54: 123–135
16. London WT, Stevens RG, Shofer FS, Drew JS, Brunhofer JE, Blumberg BS (1982) Effects of hepatitis B virus on the mortality, fertility and sex ratio of human populations. In: Szmuness W, Alter HJ, Maynard JE (eds) Viral hepatitis. Franklin Institute Press, Philadelphia, p 195–202
17. Drew JS, Blumberg BS, Robert-Lamblin J (1986) Hepatitis B virus and sex ratio of offspring in East Greenland. Human Biology 58: 115–120
18. London WT, Drew JS (1977) Sex differences in response to hepatitis B infection among patients receiving chronic dialysis treatment. Proceedings of the National Academy of Sciences USA 74: 2561–2563

Vaccination against Marek's Disease

Introduction

Marek's disease is a serious lymphoproliferative disease of the fowl which affects most organs and tissues but has an unusual predilection for peripheral nerves. The disease varies in severity ranging in extremes from the chronic disease, in which peripheral nerve involvement and paralytic signs are the most conspicuous features, to an acute fulminating disease in which multiple and diffuse lymphomata are present. Prior to the development and wide use of vaccines for the control of the disease, it was of great economic importance to the poultry industry throughout the world. In the acute form mortality of 30% of a flock was common, and in some cases mortality reached over 50%.

The disease is caused by an avidly cell-associated herpesvirus[1] which is now known to belong to a serologically closely related group which contains three serotypes[2-4]. Serotype 1 contains pathogenic Marek's disease viruses (MDV); serotype 2, mildly pathogenic or non-pathogenic MDV; and serotype 3, non-pathogenic viruses present in turkeys. Infection with MDV is ubiquitous in the domestic fowl and has been found in those feral jungle fowl that have been examined. Infection is persistent in individuals and does not preclude super-infection with a second isolate of the same or differing serotype. Flocks of domestic fowl are frequently infected with virus of both serotype 1 and serotype 2. The herpesvirus of turkeys is ubiquitous in turkey populations but has not been found to naturally infect the domestic fowl.

The discovery of the herpesvirus aetiology of Marek's disease in 1967[5] was soon followed by the development and use in the field of the first vaccine, which consisted of an attenuated pathogenic serotype 1 MDV in a cell-associated form[6,7]. This was followed by the introduction of a vaccine consisting of the herpesvirus of turkeys (HVT)[8,9]. This vaccine had advantages of growth to higher titres in cell culture and the ability to obtain cell-free virus, thus allowing vaccine to be lyophilised and distributed and used in the traditional manner. More recently a naturally apathogenic serotype 2 virus has also been used as a vaccine and has been shown to be particularly effective when mixed with HVT[10].

It is intended in this chapter to present the current knowledge on the viruses of Marek's disease relevant to their immunogenic properties and use as vaccines, together with a review of the experimental production of protective immunity, mechanisms of protection and use of vaccines in the field.

Serotypes

Isolates of MDV differ in pathogenicity and in their growth rate and plaque characteristics in cultured cells[11]. There seems to be broad agreement between the serological classification of von Bülow and Biggs[2,3], the growth characteristics of virus in vitro and pathogenicity. Thus, in general, serotype 1 strains form medium-sized plaques in cultured chicken kidney cells (CKC) and are pathogenic except for their artificially attenuated variants, which form large plaques. Type 2 strains form small plaques in CKC and comprise naturally occurring apathogenic strains. Type 3, which includes HVT strains, form large plaques in CKC (Table 2.1).

Table 2.1 Properties of some common strains of MDV and HVT

Serotype	Pathogenicity	Strain
1	Highly virulent	Md5, Md11, RB1B, ALA8
	Virulent	HPRS–16, GA, JM
	Mildly virulent (classic)	B14, VC
	Attenuated	HPRS–16/att, JM/att, Md11/75C, CVI 988
2	Not pathogenic (naturally occurring)	HPRS–24, HPRS–27, SB1, 6855
3	Not pathogenic turkey herpesvirus	FC 126, W THV–1, AC 16, HVT pa

Data from von Bülow and Biggs[2,3] and Lee and co-workers[12]

The apathogenic strains do not cause gross lesions, even when inoculated in immunosuppressed birds, although minor histological lesions consisting of lymphoid cell infiltrations have been observed in the peripheral nerves of chickens inoculated with the serotype 2 virus SB1 and HVT[13,14]. These are thought to be inflammatory lesions. There is evidence that different serotypes may be capable of establishing different virus–cell relationships in different sub-populations of lymphocytes. Pathogenic strains of serotype 1, for example, infect B cells cytolytically early after infection but establish a latent infection mainly in T cells[15]. Apparently, strains of serotypes 2 and 3 are capable of infecting different populations of lymphocytes, as suggested by the greater resistance of lymphocytes infected with type 2 virus to cytolysis by anti-Ia serum[16].

Strains of types 2 and 3 and the attenuated strains of type 1 are protective when used as vaccines, but HVT and SB1 are unable on their own to protect against some strains of MDV that have recently emerged[17,18]. These strains, which have been referred to as 'highly virulent', also belong to serotype 1 but have an increased ability to cause acute cytolytic infection in the early stages of the disease. These newly identified strains cause tumours in vaccinated and in genetically resistant birds.

Recent studies involving electrophoresis of virus-specific proteins[19], immunofluorescence using monoclonal antibodies[12] and restriction enzyme analysis of viral DNA[20,21] have supported the classification of von Bülow and Biggs[2,3]. In addition, evidence has been obtained for sub-type-specific differences using both restriction enzyme analysis and monoclonal antibodies for immunoprecipitation[22,23]. Thus, although strains of MDV and HVT can be divided into three distinct serotypes, there are intratypic differences which may be important in relation to cross-protection.

Proteins

A, B and C Antigens

Several virus-specific antigens can be detected in extracts of infected cells by the agar gel immunodiffusion test. Prominent among these is the A antigen, a major precipitating antigen released into the supernatant of cultured cells[24]. The antigen is a glycoprotein which is heterogeneous in size (54–70 kilodaltons) and charge (pI 4.5–5.5)[25-27]. There is evidence from pulse-chase experiments and from the use of inhibitors of glycosylation that the A antigen is a late gene product which arises as a 45 kilodalton (kd) polypeptide and is glycosylated to form two precursor polypeptides 57 kd and 61 kd, respectively. These are then processed, at least in part, by the addition of sialic acid to form the mature heterogeneous glycoprotein[27].

Although the A antigen is common to all serotypes, there are differences in its size and charge which are determined by the virus strain. Analysis of this protein by two-dimensional gel electrophoresis[19] allowed independent classification of strains into groups which agreed well with the serological classification[2,3].

There has been much interest in the A antigen, since it was thought to be a marker for pathogenicity. However, the existence of non-pathogenic strains that express the A antigen and of pathogenic strains that are apparently deficient in the antigen argues against this possibility. It now seems likely that the occurrence of multiple structural changes in the genome of MDV during attenuation of the virus by serial passage results in the loss of virulence and the concurrent reduction in the capacity of the virus to synthesise authentic A antigen, but that the two are not necessarily causally related.

The B antigen was studied extensively by Velicer and co-workers[28] and was shown to be a glycoprotein containing α-D-mannopyranosyl residues. In the presence of the dissociating agents 1 M urea and Brij 35, the B antigen had an apparent molecular weight of 58.28 kd. Thus, although A and B antigens are physically distinct, they cannot be totally separated on the basis of size. However, they can be differentiated on the basis of charge in the presence of urea and detergent and of the greater resistance of the B antigen to inactivation by trypsin. By use of partially purified B and C antigens it has been shown that B antigen is common to MDV and HVT and that at least two precipitating antigens (including C) are MDV (type 1)-specific[29].

Polypeptides

At least 35 MDV-specific polypeptides have been identified by two-dimensional gel electrophoresis of labelled immunoprecipitates[25]. The polypeptides range from 160 kd to less than 20 kd (Table 2.2), and comprise 17 proteins and 18 glycoproteins. Ten polypeptides have been reported to be phosphorylated[30]. It is of interest that the major virus-specific proteins expressed in lymphoblastoid cell lines are phosphoproteins and that one of them (34 kd) is encoded by

Table 2.2 Biochemical properties of MDV (CVI 988)-specific polypeptides synthesised in infected fibroblasts

Non-glycosylated polypeptide	Estimated MW (kd)	Migration behaviour*	Glycoprotein	Estimated MW (kd)	Migration behaviour*
p1	145–160	A	gp1	115	A–N
p2	145–160	A	gp2	65–85	A–N
p3	87	A	gp3	63–67	B
p4	46	N	gp4	60–80	A
p5	46	N	gp5	52–72	A–N
p6	45	N	gp6	61	B
p7	43	A	gp7	55	B
p8	38	N	gp8	50	B
p9	35	B	gp9	49	B
p10	33	N	gp10	45–55	N
p11	27	N	gp11	45–50	B
p12	25	N	gp12	44	N
p13	21	N	gp13	30–35	B
p14	<20	N	gp14	30–36	A–N–B
p15	<20	N	gp15	30	N
p16	<20	N	gp16	29	N
p17	<20	A	gp17	27	N
			gp18	24	B

*Migration relative to the heavy chain of immunoglobulin during electrophoresis in a pH gradient. A — acid; N — neutral; B — basic
From Zaane and co-workers[25] (by kind permission)

sequences within the repeat region of restriction enzyme fragments Bam H1 H and D which become modified during attenuation (Hirai, personal communication).

Structural and non-structural proteins have not been differentiated because of the difficulty in obtaining enveloped particles in cultured cells. However, the availability of monoclonal antibodies that neutralise infectivity has allowed the identification by immunoprecipitation of two mature MDV glycoproteins (gp60/63, gp49/50)[31] which are probably part of the viral envelope.

The majority of [^{35}S]-methionine-labelled proteins in extracts of MDV- and HVT-infected cells cross-react antigenically, as shown by immunoprecipitation using heterologous antisera. Moreover, both the number and size distribution of cross-reacting polypeptides appear to be the same irrespective of the serotype of the virus used for infection. Using hyperimmune antisera, Ikuta and co-workers[32] found as many as 20 cross-reacting proteins between MDV and HVT but did not examine antigens from cells infected with serotype 2. Silva and Lee[23] reached similar conclusions but could only detect the five major virus-specific proteins by immunoprecipitation with convalescent antisera. They showed, however, that all five proteins contained antigenic determinants that were common to all three serotypes. However, it was noted in both studies that more antigen was precipitated by homologous antibody than by heterologous antibody, which indicated a certain degree of strain specificity. By use of monoclonal antibody for immunoprecipitation it has been shown that virus-specific polypeptides carry multiple epitopes and that some are common to all serotypes, whereas others are type-specific[23,31]. Thus, p79 contains an epitope common to all serotypes and also a serotype-1-specific epitope. The mature envelope glycoproteins gp60/63 and gp49/52 contain at least two antigenic determinants common to type 1 and type 3 which are not shared with type 2. One of these sites interacts with neutralising antibody; the other does not. The same glycoproteins contain, in addition, an HVT-specific epitope. Similarly, p41, p38 and p24 contain type-1-specific and sub-type-specific epitopes. These results have provided further evidence for antigenic differences between serotypes. Strains may also be differentiated by the electrophoretic mobility of the following polypeptides by two-dimensional gel electrophoresis: p4, p5, p6 and gp3, gp5 and gp8[19].

Two virus-induced enzymes, presumably non-structural proteins, have been detected in infected cells: (1) a DNA polymerase which is sensitive to phosphonoacetate and phosphonoformate[33] and (2) a thymidine kinase[34]. It is of interest that the serotype 2 virus SB1 does not induce increased levels of kinase.

Genome

The DNA of MDV is a linear, double-stranded molecule approximately 175 kilobase pairs (kbp) long. It is similar in size to Epstein–Barr virus DNA but slightly larger than the DNA of herpes simplex virus and HVT. In neutral sucrose gradients, viral DNA has a sedimentation coefficient of 56S, corresponding to a molecular weight of 120×10^6 daltons[35]. There do not appear to be large differences in the size of the DNAs of different strains of serotype 1, as shown by contour length measurements of viral DNA by electronmicroscopy[36]. However, DNA of strains that have been attenuated by serial passage is larger by 2–3 kbp (see section on attenuation).

The density of MDV DNA in neutral CsCl is 1.705 g/ml, close to that of chick cell DNA[35]. This corresponds to a C+G content of 46%, assuming that the bases are unmodified. No differences in the density of the DNA of the GA, JM and C2 strains were found. However, changes in buoyant density of viral DNA occur during serial passage of virus in chick embryo fibroblasts[37]. DNA isolated from plaque-purified virus that had been cultured for 6 passages banded as a homogeneous peak (density 1.705 g/ml), whereas DNA obtained after 15 passages was heterogeneous in density and had a major peak of density 1.700 g/ml. It is not known whether these changes are the result of intramolecular rearrangements in which DNA of lower density displaces DNA of higher density in other parts of the genome.

The DNA of HVT (molecular weight 103×10^6 daltons) is smaller in size but is of higher density (1.707 g/ml) than MDV DNA. It is also linear, is double-stranded and contains 'nicks' as found for MDV DNA[38,39]. DNA of a highly passaged HVT (HVT HP) which had lost its capacity to confer protective immunity to Marek's disease appeared similar in size and in buoyant density to a vaccine strain (HVT 01) that had been passed 20 times[38]. The changes responsible for the loss of the capacity of this virus to grow in chickens are not detectable by restriction enzyme analysis, and remain to be determined.

MDV DNA has been shown to be infectious both in vitro and in vivo. The specific infectivity was 10 p.f.u./μg in chick embryo fibroblasts, and the latent period of tumour development after intra-abdominal inoculation was reported to be 6 weeks[40]. These are interesting observations, since they open up the possibility of investigating genome function by transfection with modified DNA.

The structure of MDV DNA closely resembles the DNA structure of herpes simplex virus and not that of other lymphotropic oncogenic viruses such as the EBV and herpesvirus saimiri. Electron microscopy of partially denatured DNA[36] showed that both MDV and HVT DNAs contained long and short regions of unique nucleotide sequences (U_L and U_S, respectively) each enclosed by inverted repeat sequences, as shown in Figure 2.1. There is evidence from both electron microscopy and restriction enzyme analysis that the terminal repeats are heterogeneous. Although the structure of MDV and HVT predicts that inversion of U_L and U_S could occur by intramolecular recombination, direct evidence for this by restriction enzyme analysis has not been obtained.

Libraries of cloned restriction enzyme fragments of GA, HPRS-16/att and HPRS-24 strains have been obtained, and physical maps of restriction enzyme sites of the GA virus have been constructed[41]. Three features of MDV DNA are noteworthy: (1) the presence of repeat units reminiscent of direct repeats in EBV

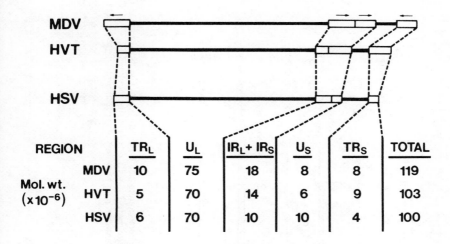

REGION	TR_L	U_L	$IR_L + IR_S$	U_S	TR_S	TOTAL
MDV	10	75	18	8	8	119
HVT	5	70	14	6	9	103
HSV	6	70	10	10	4	100

Mol. wt. $(\times 10^{-6})$

Fig. 2.1   Genome structure of MDV, HVT and herpes simplex virus (HSV) determined by electron microscopy. U_L and U_S refer to the long and short regions of unique sequences. TR_L and TR_S are the terminal repeats and IR_L and IR_S are internal repeats. Data from Cébrian and co-workers[36] (by kind permission)

DNA which divides the U_L region into two regions; (2) the presence of heterogeneous terminal fragments which are not found internally; and (3) the presence of sequences homologous to the junction of U_L and IR_L (Bg11 M fragment) throughout the viral genome.

Viruses of serotypes 1, 2 and 3 each have a unique restriction enzyme pattern[20,21,38]. There is little homology between the three serotypes as determined by reassociation kinetics experiments under stringent hybridisation conditions[20,21,42], in spite of antigenic similarities between them. In Southern blot hybridisation, only the Bam H1 J fragment of HVT formed stable hybrids with MDV DNA under stringent hybridisation conditions, and it has been estimated that the most conserved sequences are 400 bp long[43]. However, weak homology between many regions of viral DNA of the three serotypes has been demonstrated under less stringent hybridisation conditions that allow detection of homology between sequences that are 30% mismatched[22,43-45]. The results summarised in Figure 2.2 suggest that some sequences are conserved among the serotypes and that there are quantitative and qualitative differences in homology between the serotypes in different parts of the genome[22]. The presence of type-common and of type-specific epitopes on the same protein and glycoprotein molecules is consistent with this finding.

Attenuation

Serial passage of virulent virus in chicken kidney cells or in chick embryo fibroblasts results in attenuation. Comparison of the restriction enzyme patterns of

HOMOLOGY BETWEEN SEROTYPES

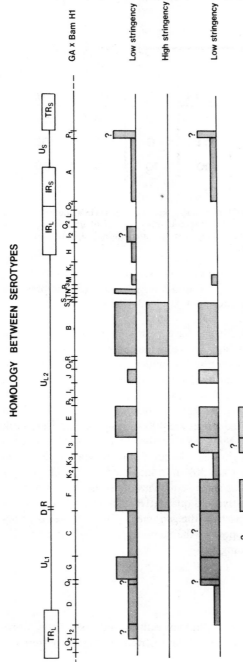

Fig. 2.2 Summary of cross-hybridisation results, showing genome map positions of homologous sequences among the three serotypes. The linkage map of Bam H1 fragments is that of Fukuchi and co-workers[41] (by kind permission). The conditions of hybridisation were $T_m - 40°C$ (low stringency) and $T_m - 24°C$ (high stringency). Histograms show relative intensity of hybridisation on an arbitrary scale. (?) indicates tentative map positions of cross-hybridising sequences. Data from Ross and co-workers[22] (by kind permission)

virulent virus strains with their attenuated derivatives shows that some restriction fragments (Bam H1 H and D and EcoR1 F)[21,46] appear to be missing in digests of attenuated virus (Fig. 2.3). Subsequent studies have shown that these fragments have increased in size during attenuation and co-migrate with other fragments[21]. These increases in fragment size have been shown to be due to an approximately tenfold expansion of a 100 bp sequence within the repeat regions

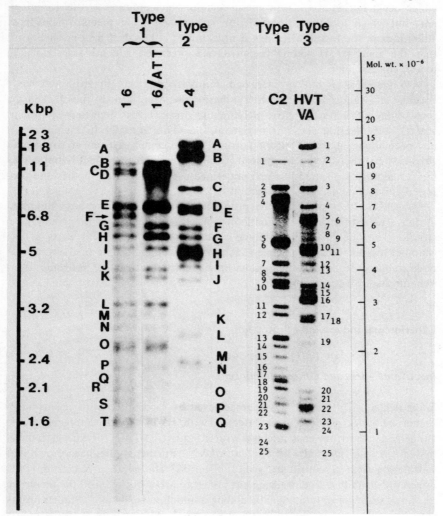

Fig. 2.3 Restriction enzyme patterns of ^{32}P-labelled DNA from several strains. Results shown are for the EcoR1 enzyme. Note that each serotype has a unique pattern and that fragment F (6.8 kbp) present in HPRS–16 appears to be missing in a digest of attenuated virus (16/att). Data from Ross and co-workers[21] and Hirai and co-workers[38] (by kind permission)

flanking the long unique sequence U_L. Similar changes have been reported in the Bam H1 A fragment which spans the internal repeat region IR_S of the short unique sequence[47].

The structural changes that have been noted during attenuation are not artifacts due to accumulation of defective DNA, since analysis of plaque-purified attenuated virus shows similar changes[22]. Thus, it appears that the changes which occur during attenuation are in regions which are not essential for infectivity but which could be important for pathogenicity. The precise role of these alterations in the loss of virulence is not known, although it may be significant that the Bam H1 H and D fragments are preserved and are transcribed in lymphoma cell lines.

Attenuated virus has an increased ability to replicate in vitro and has a considerably reduced capacity to synthesise the A antigen. In the chicken the replication of attenuated virus in lymphoid organs is less than that of virulent virus[48] and infection does not, in general, spread horizontally. In one instance it has been reported that a plaque-purified isolate obtained from an attenuated virus (JM-16) that had been passaged 55 times was unable to infect lymphocytes but apparently replicated in some undefined cells, induced antibodies and conferred a moderate degree of protection[49].

It is likely that many of the properties of virus that have been modified during attenuation are attributable to the structural changes observed by restriction enzyme analysis. As these changes occur in different parts of the genome, it is likely that multiple functions are affected. Some of these may be undesirable, especially if they occur in sequences that encode antigenic determinants associated with immunity.

Experimental Induction of Protection

Inactivated Virus and Other Immunogens

Some degree of protection has been achieved by vaccination with plasma membranes of chick embryo cells infected with HVT[50], with detergent-soluble antigens derived from cells infected with attenuated MDV[51] or with glutaraldehyde-fixed cells infected with virulent MDV[52]. Further studies have shown that vaccination with glycoproteins gp111/110, gp63 and gp50 derived from HVT-infected cells induced neutralising antibodies to MDV but reduced the incidence of Marek's disease only marginally among immunised chickens[53]. Similar results have been obtained by Wyn-Jones and Kaaden[54]. Although these results appear to diminish the importance of neutralising antibody in protection, it is possible that a greater degree of protection could be achieved by inducing higher titres of antibody for a longer period. This might be made possible by improving the immunogenicity of the antigens with the help of adjuvants. It is also not known whether the antigens given were capable of inducing cell-mediated immune responses, which are thought to be important in immunity to Marek's disease[55,56].

Protection has also been conferred by immunisation with glutaraldehyde-fixed lymphoblastoid cell lines[52]. Two inoculations with approximately 10^8 cells given with adjuvant at 16 days and without adjuvant at 39 days reduced mortality due to Marek's disease by 50%. The nature of the antigens that induced immunity in this case is not clear. Tumour-associated surface antigens (MATSA) [57,58] have been detected in cell lines by immunofluorescence using heterologous antibody raised against cell lines and absorbed with normal lymphoid cells until specific for cell lines. The gradual accumulation of MATSA-positive cells during development of the disease and their presence in lymphomas and as the majority of cells of lymphoid cell lines provide good evidence that MATSA is a marker for transformed or latently infected lymphocytes[59]. The absence of MATSA in infected fibroblasts and in Marek's disease lymphomas in other species, such as Japanese quails and bobwhite quails[60], argues against the possibility that it is virus-coded. It is thought to be a modified host-coded antigen having a molecular weight of 40 kd[61].

However, the possibility that virus-coded proteins are present in transformed lymphocytes cannot be ruled out, since selective transcription of MDV DNA and selective expression of MDV-specific phosphoproteins in cell lines have been reported[62]. It is possible that such proteins are not detectable by immuno-fluorescence using convalescent antisera, because of lack of sensitivity. Alternatively, it is possible that unknown virus-specific antigens which are unrelated to MATSA and which do not provoke antibody responses may be the target of cell-mediated immune reactions. Some support for this theory has been obtained by the demonstration that immunisation with inactivated antigens from chicken kidney cells infected with virulent MDV induced immunity to a transplantable tumour (JMV) which does not express viral antigens as shown by immuno-fluorescence[63]. In contrast, immunisation with inactivated antigens derived from fibroblasts or chicken kidney cells infected with HVT, MDV/att or SB1 failed to protect against the transplantable tumour JMV[64,65]. This suggests that there are antigens unique to virulent MDV which are important targets for rejection of tumours and that these antigens are lacking in cells infected with MDV/att, HVT and SB1.

Vaccination studies using inactivated antigens have contributed immensely to our understanding of basic mechanisms in vaccinal immunity and have laid the foundations for future generations of novel vaccines.

Vaccination in the Field

The first strain used as a vaccine was obtained by attenuation of HPRS-16 by serial passage in chicken kidney cells[6]. The HPRS-16/att vaccine, which is cell-associated, was used extensively in Europe in 1970. It has been superseded by other strains — in particular, HVT, because the latter can be lyophilised, which is attractive from a manufacturing viewpoint. Several strains of MDV were subsequently attenuated but have not been extensively used[66-68]. These artificially attenuated viruses do not spread by contact except for the CVI 988 strain[69], a mildly virulent type 1 strain which has undergone 20 passages in vitro. This cell-associated vaccine is widely used in the Netherlands, although it has been reported to be weakly pathogenic for genetically susceptible chickens[70]. Although this strain is capable of spreading by contact, the spread of infection is not rapid enough to give protection against early exposure to virulent virus. This vaccine, therefore, like the other attenuated ones, is administered as infected cells by individual inoculation of chicks at hatching[71].

Recently the attenuation of a highly virulent strain of MDV has been described[72]. This vaccine strain (Md11/75C) was particularly effective against highly virulent strains but was relatively less efficacious against challenge with JM/102W, a type 1 strain which could be effectively controlled by vaccination with HVT[72]. This suggested that vaccinal immunity is partly strain-specific. One disadvantage of the Md11/75C vaccine is that it is highly susceptible to neutralisation by homologous and heterologous maternal antibody, even in the cell-associated form.

Herpesvirus of turkeys, first isolated by Kawamura et al.[73], was shown to be non-pathogenic and antigenically related to MDV[74]. Although this virus spreads readily among turkeys, spread by contact is poor in chickens. Okazaki and co-workers[75] were the first to describe the efficacy of the FC126 strain of HVT as a vaccine. Several other strains of HVT have since been isolated which appear also to be useful as vaccines[76-78]. The HVT vaccine, which is available both as cell-associated and as cell-free viruses, has been used throughout the world for more than a decade and has been highly effective.

The efficacy of serotype 2 viruses in preventing Marek's disease was observed by Biggs and co-workers[79] and by Zander and co-workers[80]. Strains of serotype 2 which have been used as vaccines are MDV 19[68] and SB1[81]. Infectivity of serotype 2 vaccines is cell-associated in cultured cells but infection by contact occurs rapidly. The SB1 strain protects against most virulent MDV strains but was ineffective against challenge with the highly virulent strain Md5[72].

Excessive losses among broiler and layer flocks vaccinated with HVT have been noted in many countries in recent years. In the USA some of the losses are attributable to MDV strains, such as Md5 and Md11 which have been referred to as 'highly virulent'. The observation by Witter[72] that vaccinal immunity may be partly strain-specific has led to the use of mixtures of serotypes for vaccination. A trivalent vaccine consisting of an attenuated strain of the highly virulent strain Md11, and SB1 and HVT afforded better protection against a number of highly virulent strains[72,82]. Subsequently it was found that a bivalent vaccine consisting of SB1 and HVT (strain FC126) was as effective as a mixture of strains of the three serotypes in field trials on commercial broiler and layer flocks[83,84]. The mechanism of the synergistic effect is unknown, but it is conceivable that type

2 and type 3 strains could each have antigens in common with type 1 which they do not share between themselves.

In practice, vaccines are usually administered intramuscularly (2000–4000 p.f.u.) at 1 day of age. Bivalent vaccines consisting of HVT and SB1 are administered as cell-associated vaccines which are mixed immediately before inoculation. Protection against challenge may develop after 24 h, but maximal protection requires a period of at least 1 week to develop.

Mechanisms of Protection

The role of an antiviral immune response in protection is evident from the fact that immunisation with inactivated antigens derived from infected fibroblasts prevents the disease[50-52]. Antiviral immune responses comprising neutralising antibody[85], antibody-dependent cell (probably macrophage)-mediated immunity [86,87] and T-cell-mediated immunity [86,58] have been demonstrated in vaccinated birds. Although these immune responses do not prevent infection with virulent virus, the number of infected circulating lymphocytes[14,51], the spread of infection throughout the body and damage to lymphoid organs due to early cytolytic infection are considerably reduced[13,14,88]. Consequently, it is believed that vaccinated birds remain immunologically competent to reject infected and transformed lymphocytes. There is evidence that the antiviral immune response may be cell-mediated, since immunity can be conferred with inactivated MDV antigens in bursectomised birds[56]. However, a humoral immune response may be required in the case of vaccination with HVT, since sensitised lymphocytes from birds vaccinated with HVT were relatively inefficient in preventing the growth of MDV compared with sensitised lymphocytes from birds vaccinated with attenuated MDV[86]. Further support for the role of a humoral response in HVT vaccination has been obtained by bursectomy experiments which showed that birds were poorly protected in the absence of antibody. These results emphasise the differences between MDV and HVT vaccines, and suggest that homologous antigens may be better immunogens for immunisation against MDV.

An immune response against transformed lymphocytes bearing tumour-associated antigens is also operative in vaccinated birds. The antitumour immunity has been dissociated from the antiviral response, since immunisation with lymphoblastoid cell lines did not induce virus-neutralising antibody and failed to reduce lymphocyte-associated viraemia early after infection[52]. Although the nature and origin of the tumour-associated antigens is unresolved, it is clear that an antitumour immune response is important in protection, since vaccination with live vaccines prevents the growth of transplantable tumours[65,90]. The mechanism of tumour rejection is thought to be cell-mediated[91].

Macrophages probably in co-operation with antibody are able to restrict MDV replication[92] and the proliferation of lymphoid cell lines in vitro[93]. However, the role of macrophages in protection is equivocal, since they are also responsible for immunosuppression early after infection, as shown by the decreased response of spleen cells to mitogens[94]. Similar effects may be produced by normal macrophages in large numbers[95]. Nonetheless, it is possible that natural immune mechanisms involving macrophages and natural killer cells[96] contribute to protection in some non-specific manner.

Conclusions and Future

Evidence has accumulated in recent years that vaccinal immunity has an element of strain specificity and that HVT may lack antigenic determinants which are important for protection against some strains of MDV. Attenuation of the virulent strains by serial passage may not provide adequate immunity, because of multiple structural changes in the genome and the loss of antigens which participate in the rejection of transplantable tumours. These observations suggest that antigens encoded by the virulent strains are more effective immunogens than heterologous antigens and that vaccines that are effective against a whole range of virulent strains encountered in the field should be developed in the future.

Several strategies, including mutagenesis of genes associated with virulence, modification of strains of HVT by substitution of relevant MDV sequences for HVT sequences and the construction of multivalent hybrid viruses that express MDV antigens, might conceivably lead to the development of improved vaccines. However, much remains to be done to identify the genes associated with immunogenicity and oncogenicity. So far, the envelope glycoproteins involved in neutralisation of infectivity have been characterised, and sequences which may be associated with oncogenicity are being investigated.

Acknowledgements

We thank colleagues in the Microbiology Department of the Houghton Poultry Research Station, who reviewed the manuscript and made helpful comments. L.J.N. Ross is grateful to the Leukaemia Research Fund for support.

References

1. Biggs PM, Churchill AE, Rootes DG, Chubb RC (1968) The etiology of Marek's disease – an oncogenic herpes-type virus. Perspectives in Virology 6: 211–237
2. Bülow V von, Biggs PM (1975) Differentiation between strains of Marek's disease virus and turkey herpesvirus by immunofluorescence assays. Avian Pathology 4: 133–146
3. Bülow V von, Biggs PM (1975) Precipitating antigens associated with Marek's disease viruses and herpesvirus of turkeys. Avian Pathology 4: 147–162
4. Bülow V von, Biggs PM, Frazier JA (1975) Characterization of a new serotype of Marek's disease herpesvirus. In: De-Thé G, Epstein MA, Zur Hausen H (eds) Oncogenesis and herpesviruses.II. International Agency for Research on Cancer, part 2, Lyon, p 329–336

5. Churchill AE, Biggs PM (1967) Agent of Marek's disease in tissue culture. Nature 215: 528–530
6. Churchill AE, Payne LN, Chubb RC (1969) Immunization against Marek's disease using a live attenuated virus. Nature 221: 744–747
7. Biggs PM, Payne LN, Milne BS, Churchill AE, Chubb RC, Powell DG, Harris AH (1970) Field trials with an attenuated cell associated vaccine for Marek's disease. Veterinary Record 87: 704–709
8. Okazaki W, Purchase HG, Burmester BR (1970) Protection against Marek's disease by vaccination with a herpesvirus of turkeys. Avian Disease 14: 413–429
9. Purchase HG, Okazaki W, Burmester BR (1971) Field trials with the herpesvirus of turkeys (HVT) strain FC126 as a vaccine against Marek's disease. Poultry Science 50: 775–783
10. Witter RL (1984) Guest Editorial – A new strategy for Marek's disease immunization – bivalent vaccine. Avian Pathology 13: 133–135
11. Biggs PM, Milne BS (1972) Biological properties of a number of Marek's disease virus isolates. In: Biggs PM, De-Thé G, Payne LN (eds) Oncogenesis and herpesviruses. International Agency for Research on Cancer, Lyon, p 139–146
12. Lee LF, Liu X, Witter RL (1983) Monoclonal antibodies with specificity for three different serotypes of Marek's disease viruses in chickens. Journal of Immunology 130: 1003–1006
13. Calnek BW, Carlisle JC, Fabricant J, Murthy K, Schat KA (1979) Comparative pathogenesis studies with oncogenic and non-oncogenic Marek's disease viruses and turkey herpesvirus. American Journal of Veterinary Research 40: 541–548
14. Witter RL, Sharma JM, Offenbecker J (1976) Turkey herpesvirus infection in chicks: Induction of lymphoproliferative lesions and characterisation of vaccinal immunity against Marek's disease. Avian Diseases 20: 676–692
15. Calnek BW, Schat KA, Ross LJN, Shek WR, Chen CLH (1984) Further characterisation of Marek's disease virus-infected lymphocytes. I. *In vivo* infection. International Journal of Cancer 33: 389–398
16. Shek WR, Schat KA, Calnek BW (1982) Characterization of non-oncogenic Marek's disease virus-infected and turkey herpesvirus-infected lymphocytes. Journal of General Virology 63: 333–341
17. Witter RL, Sharma JM, Fadly AM (1980) Pathogenicity of variant Marek's disease virus isolates in vaccinated and unvaccinated chickens. Avian Diseases 24: 210–232
18. Schat KA, Calnek BW, Fabricant J (1982) Characterization of two highly oncogenic strains of Marek's disease virus. Avian Pathology 11: 593–605
19. Zaane D van, Brinkhof JMA, Gielkens ALJ (1982) Molecular-biological characterization of Marek's disease virus. II. Differentiation of various MDV and HVT strains. Virology 121: 133–146
20. Kaschka-Dierich C, Bornkamm CW, Thomssen R (1979) No homology detectable between Marek's disease virus (MDV) DNA and herpesvirus of the turkey (HVT) DNA. Medical Microbiology and Immunology 165: 223–239
21. Ross LJN, Milne BS, Biggs PM (1983) Restriction endonuclease analysis of Marek's disease virus DNA and homology between strains. Journal of General Virology 64: 2785–2790
22. Ross LJN, Milne BS, Schat KA (1985) Restriction enzyme analysis of Marek's disease virus DNA and homology between strains. II. In: Calnek BW, Spencer JL (eds) Proceedings of an International Symposium on Marek's disease, Cornell University, July 1984. American Association of Avian Pathologists, p 51–67
23. Silva RF, Lee LF (1984) Monoclonal antibody mediated immunoprecipitation of proteins from cells infected with Marek's disease virus and turkey herpesvirus. Virology 136: 307–320
24. Churchill AE, Chubb RC, Baxendale W (1969) The attenuation with loss of oncogenicity of the herpes-type virus of Marek's disease (strain HPRS–16) on passage in cell culture. Journal of General Virology 4: 557–564
25. Zaane D van, Brinkhof JMA, Westenbrink F and Gielkens ALJ (1982) Molecular biological characterization of Marek's disease virus. I. Identification of virus-specific polypeptides in infected cells. Virology 121: 116–132

26. Ross LJN, Biggs PM, Newton AA (1973) Purification and properties of the A antigen associated with Marek's disease virus infection. Journal of General Virology 18: 291–304

27. Ikuta K, Ueda S, Kato S, Hirai K (1983) Monoclonal antibodies reactive with the surface and secreted glycoproteins of Marek's disease virus and herpesvirus of turkeys. Journal of General Virology 64: 2597–2610

28. Velicer LF, Yager DR, Clark JL (1978) Marek's disease herpesviruses. III. Purification and characterization of Marek's disease herpesvirus B antigen. Journal of Virology 27: 205–217

29. Ross LJN, Bassarab O, Walker DJ, Whitby B (1975) Serological relationship between a pathogenic strain of Marek's disease virus, its attenuated derivative and herpesvirus of turkeys. Journal of General Virology 28: 37–47

30. Ikuta K, Nishi Y, Kato S, Hirai K (1981) Immunoprecipitation of Marek's disease virus-specific polypeptides with chicken antibodies purified by affinity chromatography. Virology 114: 277–281

31. Ikuta K, Ueda S, Kato S and Hirai K (1984) Identification with monoclonal antibodies of glycoproteins of Marek's disease virus and herpesvirus of turkeys related to virus neutralization. Journal of Virology 49: 1014–1017

32. Ikuta K, Ueda S, Kato S, Hirai K (1983) Most virus-specific polypeptides in cells productively infected with Marek's disease virus or herpesvirus of turkeys possess cross-reactive determinants. Journal of General Virology 64: 961–965

33. Reno JM, Lee LF, Boezi JA (1978) Inhibition of herpesvirus replication and herpesvirus-induced polymerase by phosphonoformate. Antimicrobial Agents and Chemotherapy 13: 188–192

34. Schat K, Schinazi RF, Calnek BW (1984) Cell-specific antiviral activity of 1-(2-fluoro-2-deoxy-β-Darabinofuranosyl)-5-iodocytosine (FIAC) against Marek's disease herpesvirus and turkey herpesvirus. Antiviral Research 4: 259–270

35. Lee LF, Kieff ED, Bachenheimer S, Roizman B, Spear PG, Burmester BR, Nazerian K (1971) Size and composition of Marek's disease virus deoxyribonucleic acid. Journal of Virology 7: 289–294

36. Cebrian J, Kaschka-Dierich C, Berthelot N, Sheldrick P (1982) Inverted repeat nucleotide sequences in the genomes of Marek's disease virus and the herpes virus of the turkey. Proceedings of the National Academy of Sciences USA 79: 555–558

37. Tanaka A, Lee YS, Nonoyama M (1980) Heterogeneous population of virus DNA in serially passaged Marek's disease virus preparation. Virology 103: 510–513

38. Hirai K, Ikuta K, Kato S (1979) Comparative studies on Marek's disease virus and herpesvirus of turkey DNA. Journal of General Virology 45: 119–131

39. Kaaden OR, Scholtz, A, Ben-Zeev A, Becker Y (1977) Isolation of Marek's disease virus DNA from infected cells by electrophoresis on polyacrylamide gels. Archives of Virology 54: 75–83

40. Kaaden OR (1978) Transfection studies in vitro and in vivo with isolated Marek's disease virus DNA. In: De-Thé G, Henle W, Rapp F (eds) Oncogenesis and herpesviruses. III. IARC Scientific Publication, part 2, p 267–268

41. Fukuchi K, Sudo M, Lee YS, Tanaka A, Nonoyama M (1984) Structure of Marek's disease virus DNA: Detailed restriction enzyme map. Journal of Virology 51: 102–109

42. Lee YS, Tanaka A, Silver S, Smith M, Nonoyama M (1979) Minor homology between herpesvirus of turkey and Marek's disease virus. Virology 93: 277–280

43. Hirai K, Ikuta K, Maotani K, Kato S (1984) Evaluation of DNA homology of Marek's disease virus, herpesvirus of turkeys and Epstein–Barr virus under varied stringent hybridization conditions. Journal of Biochemistry 95: 1215–1218

44. Gibbs CP, Nazerian K, Velicer LF, Kung HJ (1984) Extensive homology between Marek's disease herpesvirus and its vaccine virus herpesvirus of turkeys. Proceedings of the National Academy of Sciences USA 81: 3365–3369

45. Fukuchi K, Sudo M, Tanaka A, Nonoyama M (1985) Map location of homologous regions between Marek's disease virus and herpesvirus of turkey and the absence of detectable homology in the putative tumour-inducing gene. Journal of Virology 53: 994–997

46. Hirai K, Ikuta K, Kato S (1981) Structural changes of the DNA of Marek's disease virus during serial passage in cultured cells. Virology 115: 385–389
47. Fukuchi K, Tanaka A, Schierman LW, Witter RL, Nonoyama M (1985) The structure of Marek's disease virus DNA: The presence of unique non-pathogenic viral DNA. Proceedings of the National Academy of Sciences USA 82: 751–754
48. Phillips PA, Biggs PM (1972) Course of infection in tissues of susceptible chickens after exposure to strains of Marek's disease virus and turkey herpesvirus. Journal of the National Cancer Institute 49: 1367–1373
49. Schat KA, Calnek BW, Fabricant J, Graham DL (1985) Pathogenesis of infection with attenuated Marek's disease virus strains. Avian Pathology 14: 127–145
50. Kaaden OR, Dietzschold B, Ueberscher S (1974) Vaccination against Marek's disease: Immunising effect of purified turkey herpesvirus and cellular membranes from infected cells. Medical Microbiology and Immunology 159: 261–269
51. Lesnik F, Ross LJN (1975) Immunization against Marek's disease using Marek's disease virus-specific antigens free from infectious virus. International Journal of Cancer 16: 153–163
52. Powell PC, Rowell JG (1977) Dissociation of antiviral and antitumour immunity in resistance to Marek's disease. Journal of the National Cancer Institute 59: 919–924
53. Kato S, Ikuta K, Nakajima K, Ono K, Ueda S, Hirai K (1985) Analysis of virus proteins specific to and cross-reactive with Marek's disease virus and herpesvirus of turkeys using monoclonal antibodies. In: Calnek BW, Spencer JL (eds) Proceedings of an International Symposium on Marek's disease, Cornell University, July 1984. American Association of Avian Pathologists, p 111–129
54. Wyn-Jones AP, Kaaden OR (1979) Induction of virus neutralizing antibody by glycoproteins isolated from chicken cells infected with a herpesvirus of turkeys. Infection and Immunity 25: 54–59
55. Ross LJN (1977) Antiviral T cell mediated immunity in Marek's disease. Nature 268: 644–646
56. Payne LN, Powell PC, Rennie M, Ross LJN (1978) Vaccination of bursectomised chickens with inactivated Marek's disease virus-specific antigens. Avian Pathology 7: 427–432
57. Powell PC, Payne LN, Frazier JA, Rennie M (1974) T lymphoblastoid cell lines from Marek's disease lymphomas. Nature 251: 79–80
58. Witter RL, Stephens EA, Sharma JM, Nazerian K (1975) Demonstration of a tumour-associated surface antigen in Marek's disease. Journal of Immunology 115: 117–183
59. Powell PC (1985) Marek's disease virus in the chicken. In: Klein G (ed) Advances in viral oncology. Raven Press, New York, vol 5, p 103–127
60. Powell PC, Rennie M (1984) The expression of Marek's disease tumour-associated surface antigen in various avian species. Avian Pathology 13: 345–349
61. Ross LJN (1982) Characterization of an antigen associated with Marek's disease lymphoblastoid cell line MSB–1. Journal of General Virology 60: 375–380
62. Ikuta K, Nakajima K, Naito M, Soo AH, Ueda S, Kato S, Hirai K (1985) Identification of Marek's disease virus-specific antigens in Marek's disease lymphoblastoid cell lines using monoclonal antibody against virus-specific phosphorylated polypeptides. International Journal of Cancer 35: 257–264
63. Powell PC (1978) Protection against the JMV Marek's disease derived transplantable tumour by Marek's disease virus-specific antigens. Avian Pathology 7: 305–309
64. Powell PC, Rennie M (1980) Failure of attenuated Marek's disease virus and herpesvirus of turkeys antigens to protect against the JMV Marek's disease-derived transplantable tumour. Avian Pathology 9: 193–200
65. Schat KA, Calnek BW (1978) Protection against Marek's disease-derived tumour transplants by the non-oncogenic SB1 strain of Marek's disease virus. Infection and Immunity 22: 225–232
66. Spencer JL, Robertson A (1972) Influence of maternal antibody on infection with virulent or attenuated Marek's disease herpesvirus. American Journal of Veterinary Research 33: 393–400
67. Nazerian K (1970) Attenuation of Marek's disease virus and study of its properties in two different cell cultures. Journal of the National Cancer Institute 44: 1257–1267

68. Jackson CAW, Sinkovic B, Choi CO (1977) Infectivity and immunogenicity of apathogenic and attenuated Marek's disease virus vaccines. Proceedings of the 54th Annual Conference of the Australian Veterinary Association, p 149–152
69. Rispens BH, Van Vloten H, Maas HJ, Hendrick JL (1972) Control of Marek's disease in the Netherlands. I. Isolation of an avirulent Marek's disease virus strain CVI 988 and its use in laboratory vaccination trials. Avian Diseases 16: 108–125
70. Bülow V von (1977) Further characterization of the CVI 988 strain of Marek's disease virus. Avian Pathology 6: 395–403
71. Maas HJL, Borm F, Kieff G van de (1982) The prevention of Marek's disease in Holland by vaccination with cell-associated vaccines. World Poultry Science Journal 38: 163–175
72. Witter RL (1982) Protection by attenuated and polyvalent vaccines against highly virulent strains of Marek's disease virus. Avian Pathology 11: 49–62
73. Kawamura H, King DJ, Anderson DP (1969) A herpesvirus isolated from kidney cell culture of normal turkeys. Avian Diseases 13: 853–863
74. Witter RL, Nazerian K, Purchase HG, Burgoyne GH (1970) Isolation from turkeys of a cell-associated herpesvirus antigenically related to Marek's disease virus. American Journal of Veterinary Research 31: 525–538
75. Okazaki W, Purchase HG, Burmester BR (1970) Protection against Marek's disease by vaccination with a herpesvirus of turkeys. Avian Diseases 14: 413–429
76. Churchill AE, Baxendale W, Carrington G (1973) Viraemia and antibody development in chicks following the administration of turkey herpesvirus. Veterinary Record 92: 327–333
77. Zygraich N, Huygelen C (1972) Inoculation of one-day old chicks with different strains of turkey herpesvirus. I. Serological studies. Avian Diseases 16: 735–740
78. Jackson CAW, Webster AC, Van de Kooi K, Sheridan AK, Sinkovic B (1974) Field trials of herpesvirus of turkeys NSW1/70 vaccine against Marek's disease. In: Proceedings of Australian Poultry Science Conference, Hobart, Tasmania, p 238–241
79. Biggs PM, Powell DG, Churchill AE, Chubb RC (1972) The epizootiology of Marek's disease. I. Incidence of antibody, viraemia and Marek's disease in six flocks. Avian Pathology 1: 5–26
80. Zander DV, Hill RW, Raymond RG, Balch RK (1972) The use of blood from selected chickens as an immunizing agent for Marek's disease. Avian Disease 16: 163–178
81. Schat KA, Calnek BW (1978) Characterization of an apparently non oncogenic Marek's disease virus. Journal of the National Cancer Institute 60: 1075–1082
82. Witter RL, Lee LF (1984) Polyvalent Marek's disease vaccines: safety, efficacy and protective synergism in chickens with maternal antibodies. Avian Pathology 13: 75–92
83. Witter RL, Sharma JM, Lee LF, Optiz HM, Henry CW (1984) Field trials to test the efficacy of polyvalent Marek's disease vaccines in broilers. Avian Diseases 28: 44–60
84. Calnek BW, Schat KA, Peckham MC, Fabricant J (1983) Field trials with a bivalent vaccine (HVT and SB1) against Marek's disease. Avian Diseases 27: 844–849
85. Calnek BW (1972) Antibody development in chickens exposed to Marek's disease virus. In: Biggs PM, De Thé G, Payne LN (eds) Oncogenesis and herpesviruses. IARC Scientific Publications, no 2, Lyon, p 129–137
86. Ross LJN (1978) Mechanism of resistance conferred by HVT. In: Biggs PM (ed) Resistance and immunity to Marek's disease. Commission of European Communities publication, EUR 6470, Luxembourg, p 289–297
87. Kodama H, Sugimoto C, Inage F, Mikami T (1979) Anti-viral immunity against Marek's disease virus-infected chicken kidney cells. Avian Pathology 8: 33–44
88. Schierman L, Theis GA, McBride PA (1976) Preservation of a T cell-mediated immune response in Marek's disease virus infected chickens by vaccination with a related virus. Journal of Immunology 116: 1497–1499
89. Rennie M, Powell PC, Mustill BM (1980) The effect of bursectomy on vaccination against Marek's disease with the herpesvirus of turkeys. Avian Pathology 9: 557–566
90. Mason RJ, Jensen RE (1971) Marek's disease: Resistance of turkey herpesvirus infected chicks against lethal JMV agent. American Journal of Veterinary Research 32: 1625–1627

91. Sharma JM (1977) Cell-mediated immunity to tumour antigens in Marek's disease: Susceptibility of effector cells to anti-thymocyte serum and enhancement of cytotoxic activity by vibrio cholerae neuraminidase. Infection and Immunity 18: 46-51
92. Kodama H, Mikami T, Inoue M, Izawa H (1979) Inhibitory effects of macrophages against Marek's disease virus plaque formation in chicken kidney cell cultures. Journal of the National Cancer Institute 63: 1267-1271
93. Osaki K, Kodama H, Onuma M, Izawqa H, Milami T (1983) *In vitro* suppression of proliferation of Marek's disease lymphoma cell line (MDCC-MSB 1) by peritoneal exudate cells from chickens infected with MDV or HVT. Zentralblatt Veterinärmedizin 30: 223-231
94. Lee LF, Sharma JM, Nazerian K, Witter RL (1978) Suppression of mitogen induced proliferation of normal spleen cells by macrophages from chickens inoculated with Marek's disease virus. Journal of Immunology 120: 1554-1559
95. Sharma JM (1980) *In vitro* suppression of T cell mitogenic response and tumour cell proliferation by spleen macrophages from normal chickens. Infection and Immunity 28: 914-922
96. Sharma JM (1983) Presence of adherent cytotoxic cells and non-adherent natural killer cells in progressive and regressive Marek's disease tumours. Veterinary Immunology and Immunopathology 5: 125-140

Studies on the Prevention of EBV-induced Malignancies by a Sub-unit Antiviral Vaccine

Introduction

Epstein–Barr virus (EBV) was discovered 20 years ago[1]. Since that time an immense body of information has been accumulated on all aspects of the agent, and much of its general biology, molecular biology and behaviour in populations has become clear[2,3]. In the course of this work, efforts from many laboratories have established remarkably close associations between EBV and certain particular human cancers – namely, endemic Burkitt's lymphoma (BL)[4,5], the undifferentiated form of nasopharyngeal carcinoma (NPC)[6] and the lymphomas which occur in immunosuppressed allograft patients with an unusually high frequency[7-9]. The basis of these associations is well known[10-12], and recent studies on cellular oncogene activation suggest possible explanations, at least in the case of endemic BL. Thus, in endemic BL, EBV appears to play its role by infecting, and thereby 'immortalising', a pool of B lymphocytes whose virus-driven continuous cell divisions facilitate any one of three characteristic chromosomal translocations each of which can activate the c-*myc* oncogene[13]. However, since EBV is widespread in all human populations, whereas the areas where BL has a high incidence are remarkably restricted, it has long been recognised that there must be yet another element in the equation, functioning as a cofactor along with the virus and determining the geographical distribution of the endemic tumour. Suggestive epidemiological evidence has in the past been used to support the notion that hyperendemic malaria was the likely cofactor[14]. Now, firm immunological observations have demonstrated that the EBV-specific T cells which are crucial in normal circumstances for the control throughout life of EBV-infected B cells[15] show dramatically impaired function during acute attacks by *Plasmodium falciparum*[16], and, interestingly, this impairment resembles that seen in immunosuppressed renal allograft patients[17,18]. It is not difficult to envisage that in hyperendemic malarial infection, with its repeated attacks throughout the year and year after year, such impairment will favour the un-restrained growth of EBV-carrying B cells in a substantial number of individuals and thus foster the translocations and resultant c-*myc* oncogene expression, leading to a high incidence of endemic BL[13]. It should also be noted that the

HuB*lym*-1 oncogene seems to be implicated[19] in some way in this process.

Although the exact steps in the chain of events leading to the development of endemic BL are not yet fully understood, the impressive findings of the 7 year WHO prospective study in Uganda[20] make it obvious that the virus is an essential link. And within the general context of damaged EBV-specific T cell surveillance, EBV-associated lymphomas are beginning to be reported in such additional conditions of immunodepression as acquired immune deficiency syndrome (AIDS)[21]. But however the details finally turn out in endemic BL, and irrespective of whether they operate in the other EBV-related tumours, current work on the induction of lymphomas by the virus in experimental animals has shown that it alone can potently, rapidly and directly produce changes which lead to the appearance of malignant tumours[22].

The Case for a Vaccine against EBV

The foregoing introductory considerations make it clear that EBV must be regarded as having an aetiological relationship to certain malignant tumours of man. Whether this relationship reflects direct effects, as suggested by the animal experiments[22], or a more complex series of steps always involving cellular oncogenes[13], it has seemed highly likely for some time that prevention of infection by the virus would directly reduce the incidence of the associated tumours. The best analogy in this context is with carcinoma of the bronchus, where the exact carcinogenic mechanisms of cigarettes are not clear, yet it is certain that cessation of smoking in a group dramatically reduces the number of lung cancers[23]. Although the search for more and more understanding of EBV and its biological actions is of unquestionable scientific importance, it was felt already in 1976 that such efforts would be considerably enhanced in value if studies directed towards intervention against the agent were included, and the first proposals for a vaccine were therefore put forward[24].

What precedents are there for antiviral vaccination in cancer? The control of a naturally occurring herpesvirus-induced lymphoma of chickens, Marek's disease [25,26], by inoculation with attenuated or apathogenic virus[27,28], demonstrated for the first time that antiviral vaccination could dramatically reduce the frequency of a virus-induced malignant tumour (see Chapter 2). Furthermore, antigen-containing membranes from cells infected with Marek's disease herpesvirus also markedly reduced lymphoma incidence when used as an experimental vaccine[29], and even soluble viral antigens extracted from such cells protected in the same way[30]. Moving much closer to man, work with the lymphoma which can be induced in South American sub-human primates by herpesvirus saimiri[31] has shown that animals given a killed virus vaccine were protected against challenge infection and therefore did not develop tumours[32].

Requirements for an EBV Vaccine

Any vaccine for human use involving a putative oncogenic virus of man must be free of viral DNA and would best be based on an appropriate sub-unit.

A Suitable Sub-unit Antigen – MA gp340

In the EBV system the virus-neutralising antibodies developed by infected individuals are those directed against the virus-determined cell surface membrane antigen (MA)[33-36], and this information prompted the original suggestion that MA be used as an antiviral vaccine[24].

Investigations into the molecular structure of MA have identified two high-molecular-weight glycoprotein components of 340 and 270 kilodaltons (gp340 and gp270)[37-41], and the equivalence of human antibodies to MA and antibodies which neutralise EBV has been formally explained by the finding of these same glycoproteins in both the viral envelope and the cell membrane MA[40]. Not surprisingly, therefore, monoclonal antibodies which react with both MA components neutralise EBV[42,43], and gp340 and gp270 can themselves elicit virus-neutralising antibodies[44]. Most EBV-producing lymphoid cell lines synthesise roughly equal amounts of gp340 and gp270.

An Experimental Animal Model

To demonstrate the protective effects of a vaccine, it is essential to have available in the laboratory an animal capable of being infected by EBV.

Only two kinds of animal are known to be susceptible to experimental infection with the virus – the owl monkey (*Aotus*)[45-47] and the cotton-top tamarin (*Saguinus oedipus oedipus*)[48-50]. However, the former 'species' has recently been found to be very heterogeneous, with at least nine different karyotypes[51]; animals from several of these karyotypes cannot interbreed and, more important in the present context, show considerable variation in susceptibility to certain infections. The cotton-top tamarin is therefore the species of choice for experimental studies with EBV, despite having been placed on the endangered species list, for, although there was rather little information about this animal and the possibility of its successful propagation in captivity, the necessary management and husbandry conditions have now been defined[52,53]. Nevertheless, several points must be borne in mind.

1. Even though successful breeding has been achieved, cotton-top tamarins are extremely rare and very costly, and only small numbers can be used in each experiment; the constraints are similar to those operating in work on hepatitis B virus where biological tests require the use of chimpanzees.

2. Because of the constraints, it is necessary to test all methodologies with

banal laboratory animals (which can be immunised to make antibodies, for example, even though they cannot be infected with EBV) before applying them to tamarins.

3. Because of the small numbers available, any dose of virus to be administered as a challenge after vaccination must be capable of causing lesions in 100% of unprotected animals.

When young adult tamarins from the successful breeding colony were given $10^{5.3}$ lymphocyte-transforming units of EBV[54] in a large volume of fluid (7 ml) by intraperitoneal (2/3) and intramuscular (1/3) injections, lesions arose in 2-3 weeks in all the animals, and a similar rapid 100% induction of lesions has been obtained with different batches of virus in subsequent experiments; the results are summarised in Table 3.1. The lesions consisted of firm whitish masses involving lymph nodes in groins, axillae, abdomen, mediastinum and submandibular

Table 3.1   EBV-induced lymphomas in unprotected cotton-top tamarins

Experiment No.	Lymphocyte-transforming units of virus injected	Route of injection	No. of animals with lesions/ injected
1	$10^{5.3}$	iv;ip;im	2/2
2	$10^{5.3}$	ip;im	2/2
3	$10^{5.3}$	ip;im	4/4
4	$10^{5.3}$	ip;im	2/2
5	$10^{5.3}$	ip;im	4/4
6	$10^{5.3}$	ip;im	2/2

iv — intravenous
ip — intraperitoneal
im — intramuscular

regions. The nodes were enlarged from the normal 1-2 mm diameter up to 15-20 mm and were accompanied by white tumour masses (not infiltrates) in spleen, liver, kidneys, gut wall and adrenals, and filling the thoracic inlet. Each animal displayed most of these lesions and in about half of them the disease progressed; in the remaining animals the lesions regressed over 8-14 weeks, but before the onset of regression could not be distinguished clinically from those which did not. Overall, the lesions resembled those reported earlier[48-50], but appeared faster and were larger; their nature has recently been established unequivocally for the first time[22].

Histology indicated that the diseased nodes and organs were filled with large-cell malignant lymphomas of the large non-cleaved (follicular centre cell) and immunoblastic types[55]. Hybridisation studies for EBV DNA, and Southern blotting and hybridisation for immunoglobulin (Ig) gene rearrangements, showed that EBV was present in the tumours, that the apparent number of virus genomes per cell varied for individual tumours from 2 to 25, and that each tumour was composed of only one, or a few, B lymphocyte clones, as distinct from a polyclonal lymphoproliferation. Furthermore, the different tumours in the same animal arose from different cell clones.

Cell lines were established in vitro from all the tumours investigated, and were shown by Southern blotting and Ig gene probing to have arisen from the tumour cells in each case. These lines consisted of cells which expressed the EBV nuclear antigen (EBNA), and the majority shed infectious virus into the culture medium. Cytogenetic investigations failed to detect a consistent chromosomal abnormality in the cell lines. The tumours must be regarded as malignant on account of their histology and, more important, on the grounds of their monoclonality or oligo-clonality. Irrespective of whether or not subtle inapparent chromosome changes were present, the speed with which they followed inoculation of EBV makes it plain that this agent rapidly, potently and directly activated the chain of events leading to the development of multiple, different malignant tumours in each individual tamarin. Apart from their importance in vaccine studies, the tamarin tumours are also of great interest, since they seem to show a direct oncogenic role for EBV, and because they resemble in their histology, clonality and tendency to regress the EBV-related lymphomas of human allograft patients. These studies have been reported and discussed elsewhere[22].

A Sensitive Test for MA gp340

In order to work out an efficient and reliable method for the preparation of antigen, it is essential that the product can be quantified and monitored at each step to permit of modifications which maximise yields. Accordingly, a highly sensitive, quantitative radioimmunoassay (RIA) was developed for gp340, and a full account of this has been published[56].

The Efficient Preparation of MA gp340

Molecular-weight-based Method

As mentioned above, EBV-producing cell lines usually synthesise equal amounts of gp340 and gp270, but the B95-8 line[57] is anomalous in that it expresses almost exclusively the larger component, thus providing an advantage for molecular-weight-based purification. With the important help of the RIA, a preparative sodium dodecyl sulphate polyacrylamide gel electrophoresis (SDS-PAGE) procedure has been worked out for gp340 from B95-8 cells which included a new technique for ensuring that the product was renatured in an antigenic form; the details (Fig. 3.1) have already been reported[58].

Immunoaffinity Chromatography Method

gp340 has also been purified by use of a monoclonal antibody immunoabsorbent. The antigen was collected from detergent extracts of B95-8 cells on a mono-

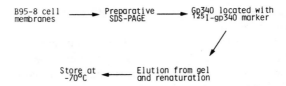

Fig. 3.1 Molecular-weight-based preparation method for MA gp340. Cell membranes from disrupted B95–8 cells were collected by centrifugation, solubilised and submitted to preparative SDS–PAGE. gp340 was located by autoradiography using highly purified [^{125}I]-gp340 as a marker, was cut out in a piece of the gel, and was eluted and separated from SDS under conditions where protein refolding was prevented by the presence of urea. The final renaturation of gp340, with good recovery of antigenicity, was brought about by removal of urea during dialysis against buffer containing non-ionic detergent[58]

clonal antibody-Sepharose column and the bound material was then eluted. The eluate, consisting of 50% gp340, was finally fractionated by gel filtration on Sephacryl, and the resulting gp340 was found to be both antigenic and 95% pure. Milligram amounts of gp340 can be obtained routinely in this way; the technical steps involved (Fig. 3.2) have all been described[59] .

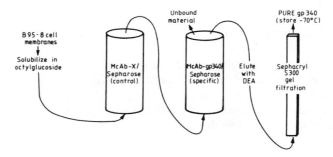

Fig. 3.2 Immunoaffinity chromatography preparation method for MA gp340. Solubilised B95–8 cell membranes, prepared as described in the caption to Figure 3.1, were applied by upward flow to an irrelevant mouse monoclonal antibody (McAb–X)/Sepharose control column to remove material which bound non-specifically, and then to a specific monoclonal antibody (McAb–gp340)/Sepharose column from which the bound material was eluted with diethylamine (DEA) and concentrated by ultrafiltration. Thereafter, the concentrated eluate was fractionated by gel filtration using upward flow through a Sephacryl S–300 column; the final gp340 product was antigenically active, 95% pure and available in milligram amounts[59]

A Potently Immunogenic MA gp340 Product

gp340 made by preparative SDS-PAGE proved only weakly immunogenic when tested in mice and rabbits by repeated injection and with the use of Freund's adjuvant. To eliminate the need for these two disadvantageous procedures, gp340 was incorporated in liposomes[60,61], sometimes with the addition of lipid

A[62], and comparative immunogenicity studies were undertaken in mice, rabbits and, later, tamarins, to determine the best routes and methods of administration. Liposomes containing gp340, with or without lipid A, gave good titres of EBV-neutralising antibodies in all three species after rather few inoculations, and all the sera were specific in that they reacted only with MA gp340 and failed to recognise any other molecule from either the surface or the interior of B95-8 cells. However, when the sera were tested against M-ABA cells[63], which also express the gp270 MA component, this antigen was recognised in addition to gp340[64], which indicates once again the sharing of antigenic determinants between the two molecules. Details of this work have been given elsewhere[44,65].

A Sensitive Assay for Antibodies to MA gp340

In order to exploit immunogenicity studies to the full, a highly sensitive test to quantify antibody responses to gp340 was required. Accordingly, a rapid enzyme-linked immunosorbent assay (ELISA) was developed, based on gp340 purified by the immunoaffinity monoclonal antibody chromatography method[59]. This ELISA has proved a thousandfold more sensitive than conventional indirect immunofluorescence tests and has made it possible to follow accurately the sequential production of specific antibodies to gp340 during the immunisation of animals. The ELISA is described in a recent publication[66].

Vaccination Experiments

The direction of the present vaccine programme has been determined from the outset by the assumption that strategies which work with the herpesvirus of Marek's disease and the lymphomas it causes in chickens would be applicable to EBV[24], an apparently carcinogenic herpesvirus of man. On this basis, EBV MA components were selected for testing as a sub-unit vaccine not only because of the concordance between human antibodies to MA and virus-neutralising anti-bodies, but also because plasma membranes from cells infected with Marek's disease herpesvirus were efficacious as an experimental vaccine in preventing infection and subsequent lymphomas in the chicken system[30]. Thus, the first and simplest step was to determine whether plasma membranes from appro-priate EBV-infected cells could be used successfully in an analogous manner.

B95-8 cells showing maximum expression of MA were disrupted, the mem-branes were collected and subjected to a sucrose-density step gradient, and the plasma membranes were then harvested at the interface (Fig. 3.3). In a pilot experiment two of the rare tamarins were immunised by intraperitoneal injection of B95-8 plasma membranes and their responses were monitored by indirect immunofluorescence, by the far more sensitive ELISA, and by standard EBV neutralisation testing which assesses the ability of a given serum to prevent

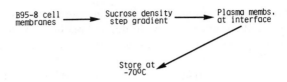

Fig.3.3 Preparation method for MA–positive plasma membranes. The membranes from disrupted B95–8 cells were collected as described in the caption to Figure 3.1 and subjected to a sucrose-density step gradient. The plasma membranes accumulated at the interface

transformation of fetal-cord blood lymphocytes by the virus[36,54]. Specific antibodies to gp340 were induced, and when these had reached high titre and were powerfully virus-neutralising (Table 3.2), the animals were challenged in the usual way with $10^{5.3}$ lymphocyte-transforming units of EBV, a dose known to induce tumours in 100% of unprotected tamarins (Table 3.1). For this significant experiment two unprotected animals were inoculated with the same material to serve as additional normal controls, and the unequivocal outcome is shown in Table 3.2. The two immunised tamarins remained entirely free of all clinically detectable lesions, whereas the normal animals developed multiple gross lesions after 2 weeks, in the same way as all other such animals before (Table 3.1).

Table 3.2 Protection of cotton-top tamarins against EBV by vaccination with B95–8 cell membranes

Tamarin	Antibody to MA (immunofluorescence)	ELISA antibody titre	Virus-neutralising antibody	Lesions after $10^{5.3}$ units of virus ip, im
Vaccinated	+++	1:800	strong*	none
Vaccinated	+++	1:2000	strong*	none
Control	–	0	none	gross
Control	–	0	none	gross

* 1 ml serum neutralised > 100 000 lymphocyte-transforming units of virus

As regards the suitability of purified gp340 as a vaccine, the demonstration that this molecule prepared by the molecular-weight-based method induced virus-neutralising antibodies in various species when injected after incorporation in liposomes was encouraging. It was therefore considered important, as the next step, to determine both the protective effect of these antibodies in tamarins, compared with those induced by plasma membranes, and the levels required for protection. A preliminary experiment of this type has been carried out: the gp340-vaccinated tamarin whose serum had potent virus-neutralising capacity was totally protected, whereas three other animals with less neutralising antibody were not[67]. A confirmatory experiment is currently well advanced and the result will be known shortly; evaluation is also under way of gp340 prepared by the immunoaffinity chromatography method. Comparison of the protection induced by inoculation of this material with that obtained using gp340 prepared by the molecular-weight-based technique should give valuable insights into the biological complexity of gp340, for the molecular-weight-based procedure theoretically isolates all epitopes on molecules of the appropriate molecular weight, whereas the monoclonal-antibody-based method is known to bind only about 50% of the MA epitopes[59]. It will be of interest to see which immunogen is most efficacious.

Discussion

With so much of the basic programme for an EBV vaccine already completed, and with the remaining aspects rapidly coming to fruition, planning for a gp340-based vaccine for man should clearly be considered sooner rather than later.

It has been emphasised in the past[24,68] that the appropriate use of this vaccine would not be in the setting of Western societies and such EBV-induced diseases as infectious mononucleosis (IM), but rather to intervene against EBV-associated endemic BL and undifferentiated NPC. The first of these two cancers is confined to rather limited areas[5,69], and in these areas other more pressing medical and community health problems take precedence. In stark contrast, however, undifferentiated NPC is the most common tumour of men and the second most common of women among Southern Chinese[6]; it has a high incidence among Eskimos[70]; and there are moderately high incidence levels in North Africa[71], East Africa[72] and through most of South East Asia[6]. The total is of considerable significance in world cancer terms. Intervention against EBV to abate undifferentiated NPC is thus a high priority.

Both endemic BL and undifferentiated NPC are diseases of developing countries, and it is well known that primary EBV infection occurs at a very early age in the social conditions and standards of hygiene of the Third World[73]. Therefore, vaccinations are required for the very young, and since undifferentiated NPC is preponderantly a disease of middle and later life[6], vaccine protection would have to be maintained for many years. However, these logistic requirements are no different from those relating to hepatitis B vaccination for the prevention of primary hepatocellular carcinoma in high-risk populations, for which plans are already well advanced (see Chapter 4).

MA components prepared in the ways discussed here[58,59] have never been thought suitable for anything beyond the present prototype vaccine[67] designed to demonstrate the capacity of these sub-units, when injected, to stimulate immunological responses giving protection against the virus. It was therefore considered important to know something of the general structure of gp340 and of the contribution, if any, of the sugar moiety of antigenicity. gp340 has been analysed after treatment with a battery of glycosidases and V8 protease, with and without preliminary exposure during synthesis to tunicamycin. This work[74] has shown that carbohydrate represents more than 50% of the total mass of gp340, that it is both O- and N-linked, that V8 protease fragments are antigenic, and that specific antibody appears to bind the protein – not the sugar. The seemingly major importance of the protein in the immunogenicity of gp340 means that for use in man the exploitation of new and sophisticated procedures can be explored.

The fragment of EBV DNA carrying the gene coding for MA has already been identified[75] and the sequence probably relating to this gene is also known[76]. Thus, the potentiality for cloning the gene and seeking to make the product by expression in suitable prokaryotic or eukaryotic cells is very real. In addition, it can be readily envisaged that the practicability of using synthetic gp340 peptides as immunogens will soon be investigated. And however the sub-unit vaccine molecule is ultimately obtained, still further possibilities lie in the direction of greatly enhancing immunogenicity by the use of powerful new adjuvants[77]. Finally, there is an excellent chance that it may prove feasible to incorporate the EBV MA gene into the genome of vaccinia virus and thus ensure its direct expression during vaccination in man[78,79].

Thus, the biological and logistic problems of an EBV vaccine intended for intervention in relation to undifferentiated NPC are no longer daunting, and the practical investigations required for such a vaccine in the human context have been recognised for some years[68]. To recall these briefly, the most advantageous situation for a trial in man is in relation to IM. Groups of young adults in Western countries can be screened to detect those who have escaped primary EBV infection in childhood and who are therefore at risk for delayed primary infection which is accompanied by the clinical manifestations of IM in 50% of cases[80,81]. This type of screening could be applied to new students entering universities or colleges and could be followed by a double-blind vaccine trial among informed, consenting volunteers in the 'at-risk' category. The effectiveness of vaccination in preventing infection and reducing the expected incidence of IM would rapidly be evident. Thereafter, the effect of vaccination and consequential prevention of disease should be assessed in a high-incidence region for endemic BL. This tumour has a peak incidence at about the age of 7, and areas with a suitably high expected number of cases are available in tropical Africa[5]; the influence of vaccination should therefore be apparent within a decade. But even while such a trial in BL was going forward, the more difficult but far more important problem of intervention against undifferentiated NPC should be addressed with the highest priority.

Acknowledgements

This work was supported by the Medical Research Council, London (Special Project Grant SPG978/32), and the Cancer Research Campaign, London (out of funds donated by the Bradbury Investment Company of Hong Kong).

References

1. Epstein MA, Achong BG, Barr YM (1964) Virus particles in cultured lymphoblasts from Burkitt's lymphoma. Lancet 1: 702–703
2. Epstein MA, Achong BG (eds) (1979) The Epstein–Barr virus. Springer, Berlin, Heidelberg, New York
3. Epstein MA, Achong BG (eds) (1986) The Epstein–Barr virus: recent advances. Heinemann, London (in press)
4. Burkitt D (1958) A sarcoma involving the jaws in African children. British Journal of Surgery 46: 218–223
5. Burkitt D (1963) A lymphoma syndrome in tropical Africa. In: Richter GW, Epstein MA (eds) International review of experimental pathology. Academic Press, New York, London, vol 2, p 67–138
6. Shanmugaratnam K (1971) Studies on the etiology of nasopharyngeal carcinoma. In: Richter GW, Epstein MA (eds) International review of experimental pathology. Academic Press, New York, London vol 10, p 361–413
7. Penn I (1978) Malignancies associated with immunosuppressive or cytotoxic therapy. Surgery 83: 492–502
8. Kinlen LJ, Sheil AGR, Peto J, Doll R (1979) Collaborative United Kingdom–Australasian study of cancer in patients treated with immunosuppressive drugs. British Medical Journal 2: 1461–1466
9. Weintraub J, Warnke RA (1982) Lymphoma in cardiac allotransplant recipients: clinical and histological features and immunological phenotype. Transplantation 33: 347–351
10. Epstein MA, Achong BG (1979) The relationship of the virus to Burkitt's lymphoma. In: Epstein MA, Achong BG (eds) The Epstein–Barr virus. Springer, Berlin, Heidelberg, New York, p 321–377
11. De-Thé G (1980) Role of Epstein–Barr virus in human diseases: infectious mononucleosis, Burkitt's lymphoma, and nasopharyngeal carcinoma. In: Klein G (ed) Viral oncology. Raven Press, New York, p 769–797
12. Klein G, Purtilo DT (eds) (1981) Epstein–Barr virus-induced lymphoproliferative diseases in immunodeficient patients. Cancer Research (Supplement) 41: 4209–4304
13. Klein G (1983) Specific chromosomal translocations and the genesis of B-cell-derived tumours in mice and men. Cell 32: 311–315
14. Burkitt DP (1969) Etiology of Burkitt's lymphoma – an alternative hypothesis to a vectored virus. Journal of the National Cancer Institute 42: 19–28
15. Rickinson AB, Moss DJ, Wallace LE, Rowe M, Misko IS, Epstein MA, Pope JH (1981) Long term T-cell-mediated immunity to Epstein–Barr virus. Cancer Research 41: 4216–4221
16. Whittle HC, Brown J, Marsh K, Greenwood BM, Seidelin P, Tighe H, Wedderburn L (1984) T cell control of B cells infected with E–B virus is lost during *P. falciparum* malaria. Nature 312: 449–450
17. Crawford DH, Sweny P, Edwards J, Janossy G, Hoffbrand AV (1981) Long-term T-cell-mediated immunity to Epstein–Barr virus in renal-allograft recipients receiving Cyclosporin A. Lancet 1: 10–13
18. Gaston JSH, Rickinson AB, Epstein MA (1982) Epstein–Barr-virus-specific T-cell memory in renal-allograft recipients under long-term immunosuppression. Lancet 1: 923–925
19. Diamond A, Cooper GM, Ritz J, Lane M-A (1983) Identification and molecular cloning of the human Blym transforming gene activated in Burkitt's lymphomas. Nature 305: 112–116
20. De-Thé G, Geser, A, Day NE, Tukei PM, Williams EH, Beri DP, Smith PG, Dean AG, Bornkamm GW, Feorino P, Henle W (1978) Epidemiological evidence for causal relationship between Epstein–Barr virus and Burkitt's lymphoma: results of the Ugandan prospective study. Nature 274: 756–761
21. Ziegler JL, Drew WL, Miner RC, Mintz L, Rosenbaum E, Gershow J, Lennette ET, Greenspan J, Shillitoe E, Beckstead J, Casavant C, Yamamoto K (1982) Outbreak

of Burkitt's-like lymphoma in homosexual men. Lancet 2: 631–633

22. Cleary ML, Epstein MA, Finerty S, Dorfman RF, Bornkamm GW, Kirkwood JK, Morgan AJ, Sklar J (1985) Individual tumours of multifocal EB virus-induced malignant lymphomas in tamarins arise from different B cell clones. Science 228: 722–724

23. Doll R, Peto R (1976) Mortality in relation to smoking: 20 years' observation on male British doctors. British Medical Journal 2: 1525–1536

24. Epstein MA (1976) Epstein–Barr virus – is it time to develop a vaccine program? Journal of the National Cancer Institute 56: 697–700

25. Marek J (1907) Multiple Nervenentzündung (Polyneuritis) bei Hühnern. Deutsche tierärztliche Wochenschrift 15: 417–421

26. Payne LN, Frazier JA, Powell PC (1976) Pathogenesis of Marek's disease. In: Richter GW, Epstein MA (eds) International review of experimental pathology. Academic Press, New York, San Francisco, London, vol 16, p 59–154

27. Churchill AE, Payne LN, Chubb RC (1969) Immunization against Marek's disease using a live attenuated virus. Nature 221: 744–747

28. Okazaki W, Purchase HG, Burmester BR (1970) Protection against Marek's disease by vaccination with a herpesvirus of turkeys. Avian Diseases 14: 413–429

29. Kaaden OR, Dietzschold B (1974) Alterations of the immunological specificity of plasma membranes of cells infected with Marek's disease and turkey herpesviruses. Journal of General Virology 25: 1–10

30. Lesnick, F, Ross LJN (1975) Immunization against Marek's disease using Marek's disease virus-specific antigens free from infectious virus. International Journal of Cancer 16: 153–163

31. Meléndez LV, Hunt RD, Daniel MD, Garcia FG, Fraser CEO (1969) Herpesvirus Saimiri. II. An experimentally induced primate disease resembling reticulum cell sarcoma. Laboratory Animal Care 19: 378–386

32. Laufs R, Steinke H (1975) Vaccination of non-human primates against malignant lymphoma. Nature 253: 71–72

33. Pearson G, Dewey F, Klein G, Henle G, Henle W (1970) Relation between neutralization of Epstein–Barr virus and antibodies to cell-membrane antigens induced by the virus. Journal of the National Cancer Institute 45: 989–995

34. Pearson, G, Henle G, Henle W (1971) Production of antigens with Epstein–Barr virus in experimentally infected lymphoblastoid cell lines. Journal of the National Cancer Institute 46: 1243–1250

35. Gergely L, Klein G, Ernberg I (1971) Appearance of Epstein–Barr virus-associated antigens in infected Raji cells. Virology 45: 10–21

36. De Schryver A, Klein G, Hewetson J, Rocchi G, Henle W, Henle G, Moss DJ, Pope JH (1974) Comparison of EBV neutralization tests based on abortive infection or transformation of lymphoid cells and their relation to membrane reactive antibodies (anti MA). International Journal of Cancer 13: 353–362

37. Qualtière LF, Pearson GR (1979) Epstein–Barr virus-induced membrane antigens: immunochemical characterisation of Triton X100 solubilised viral membrane antigens from EBV-superinfected Raji cells. International Journal of Cancer 23: 808–817

38. Strnad BC, Neubauer RH, Rabin H, Mazur RA (1979) Correlation between Epstein–Barr virus membrane antigen and three large cell surface glycoproteins. Journal of Virology 32: 885–894

39. Thorley-Lawson DA, Edson CM (1979) The polypeptides of the Epstein–Barr virus membrane antigen complex. Journal of Virology 32: 458–467

40. North JR, Morgan AJ, Epstein MA (1980) Observations on the EB virus envelope and virus-determined membrane antigen (MA) polypeptides. International Journal of Cancer 26: 231–240

41. Qualtière LF, Pearson GR (1980) Radioimmune precipitation study comparing the Epstein–Barr virus membrane antigens expressed on P_3HR-1 virus-superinfected Raji cells to those expressed on cells in a B95–8 virus-transformed producer culture activated with tumour-promoting agent (TPA). Virology 102: 360–369

42. Hoffman GJ, Lazarowitz SG, Hayward DS (1980) Monoclonal antibody against a 250,000-dalton glycoprotein of Epstein–Barr virus identifies a membrane antigen

and a neutralizing antigen. Proceedings of the National Academy of Sciences USA 77: 2979–2983

43. Thorley-Lawson DA, Geilinger K (1980) Monoclonal antibodies against the major glycoprotein (gp350/220) of Epstein–Barr virus neutralise infectivity. Proceedings of the National Academy of Sciences USA 77: 5307–5311

44. North JR, Morgan AJ, Thompson JL, Epstein MA (1982) Purified EB virus gp340 induces potent virus-neutralizing antibodies when incorporated in liposomes. Proceedings of the National Academy of Sciences USA 79: 7504–7508

45. Epstein MA, Hunt RD, Rabin H (1973) Pilot experiments with EB virus in owl monkeys (*Aotus trivirgatus*). I. Reticuloproliferative disease in an inoculated animal. International Journal of Cancer 12: 309–318

46. Epstein MA, Rabin H, Ball G, Rickinson AB, Jarvis J, Meléndez LV (1973) Pilot experiments with EB virus in owl monkeys (*Aotus trivirgatus*). II. EB virus in a cell line from an animal with reticuloproliferative disease. International Journal of Cancer 12: 319–332

47. Epstein MA, Zur Hausen H, Ball G, Rabin H (1975) Pilot experiments with EB virus in owl monkeys (*Aotus trivirgatus*). III. Serological and biochemical findings in an animal with reticuloproliferative disease. International Journal of Cancer 15: 17–22

48. Shope T, Dechairo D, Miller G (1973) Malignant lymphoma in cotton-top marmosets after inoculation with Epstein–Barr virus. Proceedings of the National Academy of Sciences USA 70: 2487–2491

49. Miller G, Shope T, Coope D, Waters L, Pagano J, Bornkamm GW, Henle W (1977) Lymphoma in cotton-top marmosets after inoculation with Epstein–Barr virus: tumour incidence, histologic spectrum, antibody responses, demonstration of viral DNA, and characterization of viruses. Journal of Experimental Medicine 145: 948–967

50. Miller G (1979) Experimental carcinogenicity by the virus *in vivo*. In: Epstein MA, Achong BG (eds) The Epstein–Barr virus. Springer, Heidelberg, New York, p 351–372

51. Ma NSF (1981) Chromosome evolution in the owl monkey, *Aotus*. American Journal of Physical Anthropology 54: 293–303

52. Kirkwood JK, Epstein MA, Terlecki AJ (1983) Factors influencing population growth of a colony of cotton-top tamarins. Laboratory Animals 17: 35–41

53. Kirkwood JK (1983) Effects of diet on health, weight and litter size in captive cotton-top tamarins *Saguinus oedipus oedipus*. Primates 24: 515–520

54. Moss DJ, Pope JH (1972) Assay of the infectivity of Epstein–Barr virus by transformation of human leucocytes *in vitro*. Journal of General Virology 17: 233–236

55. Dorfman RF, Burke JS, Berard C (1982) A working formulation of non-Hodgkin's lymphomas: background recommendations, histological criteria and relationship to other classifications. In: Rosenberg S, Kaplan H (eds) Malignant lymphomas. Academic Press, New York, p 351–368

56. North JR, Morgan AJ, Thompson JL, Epstein MA (1982) Quantification of an EB virus-associated membrane antigen (MA) component. Journal of Virological Methods 5: 55–65

57. Miller G, Shope T, Lisco H, Stitt D, Lipman M (1972) Epstein–Barr virus: transformation, cytopathic changes, and viral antigens in squirrel monkey and marmoset leukocytes. Proceedings of the National Academy of Sciences USA 69: 383–387

58. Morgan AJ, North JR, Epstein MA (1983) Purification and properties of the gp340 component of Epstein–Barr (EB) virus membrane antigen (MA) in an immunogenic form. Journal of General Virology 64: 455–460

59. Randle BJ, Morgan AJ, Stripp SA, Epstein MA (1985) Large-scale purification of Epstein–Barr virus membrane antigen gp340 using a monoclonal immunoabsorbent. Journal of Immunological Methods 77: 25–36

60. Morein B, Helenius A, Simons K, Pettersson R, Kääriäinen L, Schirrmacher V (1978) Effective subunit vaccines against an enveloped animal virus. Nature 276: 715–718

61. Manesis EK, Cameron CH, Gregoriadis G (1979) Hepatitis B surface antigen-containing liposomes enhance humoral and cell-mediated immunity to the antigen. FEBS Letters 102: 107–111

62. Naylor PT, Larsen HL, Huang L, Rouse BT (1982) *In vivo* induction of anti-herpes simplex virus immune response by Type 1 antigens and Lipid A incorporated into liposomes. Infection and Immunity 36: 1209–1216

63. Crawford DH, Epstein MA, Bornkamm GW, Achong BG, Finerty S, Thompson JL (1979) Biological and biochemical observations on isolates of EB virus from the malignant epithelial cells of two nasopharyngeal carcinomas. International Journal of Cancer 24: 294–302

64. Epstein MA, Morgan AJ (1984) Oncogenic role of Epstein–Barr virus: progress towards subunit vaccine. In: Goldman JM, Jarrett O (eds) Mechanisms of viral leukaemogenesis. Leukaemia and lymphoma research. Churchill Livingstone, Edinburgh, London, Melbourne, New York vol 1, p 184–206

65. Morgan AJ, Epstein MA, North JR (1984) Comparative immunogenicity studies on Epstein–Barr (EB) virus membrane antigen (MA) with novel adjuvants in mice, rabbits and cotton-top tamarins. Journal of Medical Virology 13: 281–292

66. Randle BJ, Epstein MA (1984) A highly sensitive enzyme-linked immunosorbent assay to quantitate antibodies to Epstein–Barr virus membrane antigen gp340. Journal of Virological Methods 9: 201–208

67. Epstein MA (1984) A prototype vaccine to prevent Epstein–Barr (EB) virus-associated tumours. Proceedings of the Royal Society of London, B 221: 1–20

68. Epstein MA (1979) Vaccine control of EB virus-associated tumours. In: Epstein MA, Achong BG (eds) The Epstein–Barr virus. Springer, Berlin, Heidelberg, New York, p 440–448

69. Ten Seldam REJ, Cooke R, Atkinson L (1966) Childhood lymphoma in the territories of Papua and New Guinea. Cancer 19: 437–446

70. Lanier A, Bender T, Talbot M, Wilmeth S, Tschopp C, Henle W, Henle G, Ritter D, Terasaki P (1980) Nasopharyngeal carcinoma in Alaskan Eskimos, Indians and Aleuts: a review of cases and study of Epstein–Barr virus, HLA and environmental risk factors. Cancer 46: 2100–2016

71. Cammoun M, Hoerner GV, Mourali N (1974) Tumors of the nasopharynx in Tunisia: an anatomic and clinical study based on 143 cases. Cancer 33: 184–192

72. Clifford P (1970) *A review*: on the epidemiology of nasopharyngeal carcinoma. International Journal of Cancer 5: 287–309

73. Henle W, Henle G (1979) Seroepidemiology of the virus. In: Epstein MA, Achong BG (eds) The Epstein–Barr virus. Springer, Berlin, Heidelberg, New York, p 61–78

74. Morgan AJ, Smith AR, Barker RN, Epstein MA (1974) A structural investigation of the Epstein–Barr (EB) virus membrane antigen glycoprotein, gp340. Journal of General Virology 65: 397–404

75. Hummel M, Thorley-Lawson DA, Kieff E (1984) An Epstein–Barr virus DNA fragment encodes messages for the two major envelope glycoproteins (gp350/300 and gp220/200). Journal of Virology 49: 413–417

76. Biggin M, Farrell PJ, Barrell BG.(1984) Transcription and DNA sequence of the *Bam*HI L fragment of B95-8 Epstein–Barr virus. EMBO Journal 3: 1083–1090

77. Morein B, Sundquist B, Höglund S, Dalsgaard K, Osterhaus A (1984) ISCOM, a novel structure for antigenic presentation of membrane proteins from enveloped viruses. Nature 308: 457–460

78. Smith GL, Mackett M, Moss B (1983) Infectious vaccinia virus recombinants that express hepatitis B virus surface antigen. Nature 302: 490–495

79. Moss B, Smith GL, Gerin JL, Purcell RH (1984) Live recombinant vaccinia virus protects chimpanzees against hepatitis B. Nature 311: 67–69

80. Niederman JC, Evans AS, Subrahmanyan L, McCollum RW (1970) Prevalence, incidence and persistence of EB virus antibody in young adults. New England Journal of Medicine 282: 361–365

81. University Health Physicians and PHLS Laboratories (1971) Infectious mononucleosis and its relationship to EB virus antibody. British Medical Journal iv: 643–646

Prevention of Primary Liver Cancer by Hepatitis B Vaccines

Introduction

Viral hepatitis is recognised as a major public health problem in all parts of the world. The term 'human viral hepatitis' refers to infections caused by four or more different viruses or groups of viruses: hepatitis A, hepatitis B; the more recently identified forms of hepatitis, non-A, non-B hepatitis, which are caused by more than two viruses and probably by several different viruses; epidemic non-A hepatitis (previously referred to as epidemic non-A, non-B hepatitis); and the delta virus. Hepatitis A and hepatitis B can be differentiated by sensitive laboratory tests for specific antigens and antibodies, and the viruses have been characterised. Specific laboratory tests are also available for the delta agent, a defective virus, which replicates in individuals infected with hepatitis B virus.

The Biology of Hepatitis B Virus

Structural and Antigenic Analysis of the Virus

Examination by electron microscopy of plasma containing hepatitis B surface antigen reveals the presence of small spherical particles measuring on average 22 nm in diameter, tubular forms of varying length but with a diameter close to 22 nm, and large double-shelled or solid particles approximately 42 nm in diameter (Fig. 4.1). The 42 nm particle is the complete virion, and contains a core or nucleocapsid about 27 nm in diameter surrounded by an envelope approximately 14 nm in thickness. The core contains a double-stranded circular DNA with a molecular weight of about 2.3×10^6. The DNA is approximately 3200 nucleotides in length, with a single-stranded gap varying from 600 to 2100 nucleotides. The core particle also contains a DNA-dependent DNA polymerase, which is closely associated with the DNA template, and protein kinase which phosphorylates the major viral specified core polypeptides. Hepatitis B *e* antigen is another antigen which is closely associated with the core and its antigenic

47

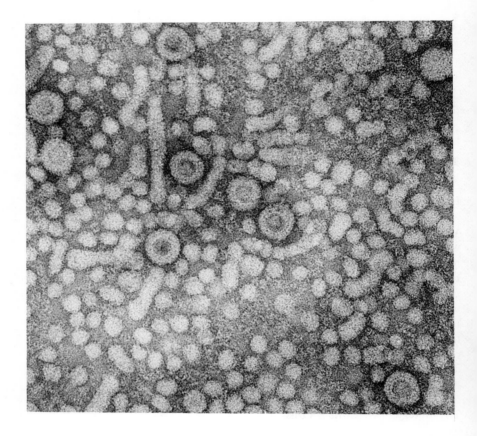

Fig. 4.1 Electron micrograph of serum showing the three morphological entities of hepatitis B: small pleomorphic spherical particles of the surface antigen, approximately 22 nm in diameter; tubular forms; and double-shelled and solid particles of the complete hepatitis B virus, approximately 42 nm in diameter, consisting of a core, about 27 nm in diameter, with a thin shell, and an outer lipoprotein coat, the surface antigen. × 252 000

reactivity. The core antigen can be converted into *e* antigen by proteolytic degradation under dissociating conditions. The small 22 nm particles and the tubular forms found in the plasma are non-infectious surplus protein of the virus coat, which also contain a variable amount of lipid and carbohydrate.

There is evidence which suggests the presence of specific structural receptors for polyalbumin on the complete virion and on purified hepatitis B surface antigen particles and polypeptides, particularly if derived from *e*-antigen-positive plasma. Polyalbumin receptors are also present on the surface of hepatocytes, with polymerised serum albumin acting as a linker molecule between the surface antigen and the cell. The virion polyalbumin receptors are species- and ligand-specific and they react only with polymerised serum albumin, whereas the hepatocyte-associated polyalbumin receptors are not ligand-specific and they react with polymeric and monomeric albumins from different species. The polyalbumin receptors are probably encoded by the genome of the hepatitis B virus.

After the virus attaches to the surface of the hepatocyte, penetration of the virus into the cell may occur by two mechanisms: endocytosis of intact virions, with subsequent release from endosomes, or fusion between the viral envelope and the liver cell plasma membrane, with penetration of the nucleocapsid into the cytoplasm. Replication of the virus in liver cells results in the production of viral proteins and the assembly of the complete virion. Hepatitis B surface antigen and core antigen are expressed on the plasma membrane of infected cells, and subsequently large amounts of the surface antigen and virus are released into the circulation.

The results of studies using monoclonal antibodies suggest that there are distinct determinants which reside on a domain common to all sub-types, but that there are also quantitative and qualitative differences in epitope density among the various sub-sets, implying that the surface antigen particles are much more heterogeneous than described hitherto. Therefore, it is now possible to 'finger-print' hepatitis B virus, which will permit of fine analysis of the evolution of the virus and its epidemiology in different parts of the world.

Immune Response to Acute Infection with Hepatitis B Virus

Infection leads to the appearance in the plasma during the incubation period of hepatitis B surface antigen about 2–8 weeks before biochemical evidence of liver dysfunction or the onset of jaundice. The surface antigen persists during the acute illness and is usually cleared from the circulation during convalescence. Viral DNA polymerase associated with the core of the virus is the next marker to appear in the circulation, at about the same time another antigen, the e antigen, becomes detectable, again preceding serum aminotransferase elevations. The e antigen is a distinct soluble antigen which correlates closely with the number of virus particles and relative infectivity. Antibody to the hepatitis core antigen is found in the serum 2–4 weeks after the appearance of the surface antigen, and it is always detectable during the early acute phase of the illness. Core antibody of the IgM class usually becomes undetectable within some months of the onset of uncomplicated acute infection, but IgG core antibody persists after recovery for many years and possibly for life. The next antibody to appear in the circulation is directed against the e antigen, and there is evidence that anti-e indicates relatively low infectivity of serum, although a better measure of infectivity is the presence of hepatitis B virus DNA in serum. Antibody to the surface antigen, hepatitis B surface antibody (anti-HBs), is the last marker to appear late during convalescence. Precipitating antibodies reacting with antigenic determinants on the complete virus particle have also been described, and these antibodies may be important for the clearance of circulating hepatitis B virions.

More recent findings indicate that at the time of replication of hepatitis B virus, the surface antigen and core antigen are expressed on the plasma membrane of infected liver cells and both cellular and immune responses are initiated. The release of large amount of surface antigen into the circulation which follows may induce high tolerance and rapid disappearance of the immune response to this antigen. Virions carrying polyalbumin receptors also stimulate the formation of neutralising polymerised human serum albumin antibodies, which prevent attachment and penetration of the virus into uninfected liver cells by reacting with the core antigen on the surface of liver cells. Thus, elimination of the virus depends on a combined cellular and humoral response, with both receptor neutralising polymerised human serum albumin antibodies and effective cytotoxic T cells. Failure of either of these mechanisms would lead to chronic liver damage and viral persistence. The extent of liver damage then depends on a number of factors, which include autoimmune reactions directed at native hepatocyte membrane antigens and modulation of lysis by T cells of infected hepatocytes expressing core antigen on the surface of the cells. This would result eventually in termination of active viral replication with seroconversion to anti-*e*, with clinical and histological remission. On the other hand, cells with integrated viral genome do not have core antigen expressed on their surface and are protected from T-cell lysis. The destruction of hepatocytes containing integrated hepatitis B virus DNA may be dependent on an immune response to hepatitis B surface antigen, and failure of this process of elimination results in persistence of clones of cells with the potential for transformation.

Hepatitis B Virus and Hepatocellular Carcinoma

Hepatocellular carcinoma is one of the ten most common cancers in the world and one of the most prevalent cancers in developing countries, with over 250 000 new cases of liver cancer each year[1]. The actual age-adjusted incidence of hepatocellular carcinoma is over 30 new cases per 100 000 population each year in some parts of Asia and Africa, whereas it is less than 5 new cases per 100 000 per year in most countries in Europe and North America and in Australia. Nevertheless, there appears to be an upward time trend in the majority of the low-incidence countries. Primary liver cancer is more common in males than among females, and it is well established that the incidence of liver cancer increases with age, but in high-risk populations the disease occurs in younger age groups. There is a marked increase in incidence in certain ethnic groups[1].

Epidemiological Correlation between Hepatitis B Infection and Hepatocellular Carcinoma

Many studies in different parts of the world, particularly in Africa and Asia, show a highly significant excess of surface antigen, core antibody and surface antibody in patients with hepatocellular carcinoma (see References 1-4 for review). An important factor in the aetiological association between hepatitis B and liver cell carcinoma may lie in an early age of infection[5,6]. In areas of the world where the prevalence of macronodular cirrhosis and hepatocellular carcinoma is high, infection with hepatitis B virus and development of the persistent carrier state occur most frequently in infants and children[7].

Production of Hepatitis B Surface Antigen by Continuous Cell Lines Derived from Human Hepatocellular Carcinoma

The establishment of continuous cell lines which produce hepatitis B surface antigen from hepatocellular carcinoma provided a laboratory model for the study of various aspects of the biology of hepatitis B. The first of these cell lines, the PLC/PRF/5 cell line, produces hepatitis B surface antigen[8] similar in size, morphology and polypeptide composition to the form which occurs in the serum of naturally infected individuals[9]. The second hepatitis B surface antigen-producing cell line, Hep 3B, which differs in some ways from the PLC/PRF/5 cells[10]. A third hepatocellular carcinoma cell line, DELSH-5, releases hepatitis B surface antigen into the medium from the thirteenth passage onwards and, like the Hep 3B cells, the cells synthesised albumin and α-fetoprotein[11]. Other similar cell lines have been derived in other laboratories.

Desmyter et al.[12] induced tumours in 80% or more of nude mice (Pfd: NMRI/*nu-nu*) injected subcutaneously in the neck with 5-10 × 10^6 cells. The tumours usually became evident after 2 weeks and grew to a size of up to 15-30% of the body weight of the mice. Metastases were not observed. When the cells were inoculated intraperitoneally, multiple tumours developed in various abdominal organs. The histology of the tumours was that of a well-differentiated human hepatocellular carcinoma. Hepatitis B surface antigen was demonstrated by immunofluorescence in 0.1-10% of the tumour cells. Hepatitis B surface antigen, but no other serological marker of hepatitis B virus, was found in the serum of the tumour-bearing mice. Newborn and weanling nude mice were found to be equally susceptible. The tumours were serially transplantable three to five times, but the tumour 'take rates' decreased with each passage, although there were not obvious differences between first-passage and later-passage tumours. The take rates were better when pieces of tumour were transplanted rather than trypsinised tumour cells. It was also possible to clone cells from the tumours, and their progeny induced tumours.

Similar tumours were obtained in nude, athymic rats (Rowerr Pfd: WIST-*rnu-rnu*), although the rats were less susceptible than nude mice. Similar results have been reported by other investigators.

Mode of Replication of Hepatitis B Virus

The inability to cultivate hepatitis B virus in vitro, the difficulties of obtaining suitable liver tissue, and, until recently, the lack of suitable experimental systems and techniques, hindered the investigation of the mode of replication of hepatitis B virus. Summers and Mason[13] proposed, on the basis of studies of the duck hepatitis B virus, that the replication cycle of hepatitis B-like viruses is strikingly different from that of other DNA viruses in that RNA-directed DNA synthesis plays an essential role in the life-cycle of these viruses, which suggests a close similarity to the RNA retroviruses. The principal unusual feature is the use of an RNA copy of the genome as an intermediate for the replication of the DNA genome. Infecting DNA genomes are converted to the double-stranded form, which serve as a template for transcription of RNA. Multiple RNA transcripts are then synthesised from each infecting genome, and these transcripts have either messenger function or DNA replicative function. The term 'pre-genomes' has been used for the transcripts with DNA replicative function; since these are precursors of the progeny DNA genomes, they are assembled into nucleocapsid and reverse-transcribed before coating and release from the cell. Each mature virus particle contains, therefore, a DNA copy of the RNA pre-genome and a DNA polymerase.

The pre-genome appears to be a single polyadenylated viral specific plus-strand RNA of approximately one genome in length (3 kb). The first DNA to be synthesised is a minus strand, and it is initiated at a unique site on the viral genome. Very small nascent DNA minus strands, as short as 30 nucleotides in length, are covalently attached at the 5' end of the minus strand to a protein, and the protein probably serves as a primer for the synthesis of the minus-strand DNA. Growth of the minus strands is accompanied by degradation of the pre-genome, so that a full-length single-stranded DNA is produced (although hybrid DNA–RNA molecules have also been reported more recently). Plus-strand DNA synthesis has been found after completion of the minus strand, and it is initiated at a unique site a few hundred nucleotides from the 5' end of the minus strand. However, complete elongation of the plus strand is not required for coating and release of the nucleocapsid cores, so that most extracellular virions contain incomplete plus strand and a single-stranded gap in the genome.

On the basis of this mode of replication, the ability of an infected cell to produce virus will depend on the continuous presence of a transcriptionally active form of viral DNA or 'proviral' DNA. The 'proviral' DNA must be present continuously, since each pregenomic RNA molecule can give rise to only one virus particle.

Weiser and co-workers[14] characterised the major forms of intracellular virus-specific DNA in the livers of experimentally infected ground squirrels. A variety of DNA structures have been found: covalently closed circular molecules, relaxed circular molecules and a heterogeneous collection of molecules associated with protein and containing minus strands in 8–10-fold mass excess of plus strands.

These results are in agreement with the analysis of intracellular forms of the duck hepatitis B virus[13].

Fowler et al.[15] characterised the DNA replicative intermediates of hepatitis B virus present in the liver of a human and chimpanzee carriers. The viral DNA forms consisted of a full-length 3.2 kb double-stranded hepatitis B viral DNA in both linear and relaxed circles; partially double-stranded DNA species of hetero-geneous length and with mobility in the range of 2.8–2.0 kb; and single-stranded DNA of heterogeneous length, with mobilities relative to double-stranded DNA of 1.6 kb and less, exclusively in the form of minus-strand DNA. The 3.2 kb double-stranded and single-stranded DNA species are considered to be replicative intermediates, since, unlike the partially double-stranded species, they are not found in hepatitis B DNA obtained from plasma. This pattern of single-stranded replicative intermediates exclusively in the form of DNA minus strands is incon-sistent with a semiconservative mechanism of DNA replication and is more like the mechanism of asymmetric replication using reverse transcription of an RNA pre-genome, as described above.

Distinct hybrid DNA–RNA molecules have been found in virus particles obtained from the plasma and liver of persistently infected patients and the liver of infected ducks. Examination of the hybrid molecules revealed the presence of viral minus-strand DNA hydrogen bonded to plus-strand RNA[16]. Localisation of hepatitis B viral DNA predominantly in the cytoplasm of liver cells by an in-situ hybridisation technique by Burrell et al.[17], and the presence in the liver of a patient with chronic active hepatitis B of mainly minus-stranded viral DNA in the cytoplasm of hepatocytes using in-situ hybridisation and by Southern blot analysis are in agreement with the view of replication of three of the hepadna viruses reported to date are remarkably similar and differ from that known for all other DNA viruses.

Integration of Hepatitis B Viral DNA in the PLC/PRF/5 Cell Line

The PLC/PRF/5 cell contains approximately four copies of viral DNA per haploid, mammalian cell DNA equivalent. There is evidence that DNA from all regions of the viral genome is present in these cells, which suggests that the cells contain most, and possibly all, of the viral genome. Furthermore, the results indicated that the viral DNA is integrated in high-molecular-weight DNA at three different sites in the cells and that there is no viral DNA in an episomal form. Cellular RNA radiolabelled with ^{32}P was found to hybridise with all restriction fragments of hepatitis B virus DNA, which suggests that most, and possibly all, of the viral DNA in these cells is transcribed.

There is also evidence for integration of the DNA of hepatitis B virus into the host genome of the PLC/PRF/5 cells and for expression of three RNA molecules containing specific sequences of hepatitis B virus. Integration of viral DNA in the cellular genome of human hepatocellular carcinoma tissue and in the PLC/PRF/5 cell line has also been demonstrated. The results suggest the existence of a limited number of integration sites in the cellular DNA, which is consistent either with the development of the liver tumour from one clone with several integration sites or with its development from a few clones each having particular integration sites. Other observations suggest the presence of two or more viral genomes inserted in tandem head-to-tail.

Integration of Hepatitis B Virus DNA into the Genome of Liver Cells

Hepatitis B virus DNA has also been found in hepatocellular carcinoma tissue. However, there is no simple correlation between serum markers of hepatitis B infection and viral DNA in the tumour. In addition, in some specimens of liver tissue adjacent to tumours, extrachromosomal and integrated viral DNA were present. The presence of integrated DNA in non-tumour tissue from patients with hepatocellular carcinoma suggests that integration precedes the development of neoplasia.

In most carriers of hepatitis B virus with a relatively recent history of liver disease and with or without histological evidence of chronic liver disease, integrated DNA has not been found. However, in several patients who were persistent carriers there was diffuse hybridisation in the high-molecular-weight regions of the gel. Free viral DNA was not identified. In these patients it is possible that viral DNA is integrated diffusely throughout the host genome. Such integration might precede a stage in persistent infection with hepatitis B virus during which a specific sub-population of hepatocytes undergoes cellular division into a clonal focus containing integrated viral DNA in one of a few specific sites. Additional factors may then be involved in the development of neoplasia from such a clonal focus.

Brechot et al.[18] used the Southern blot transfer-hybridisation technique to examine tissue-extracted DNA immobilised on nitrocellulose paper by hybridisation with cloned hepatitis B virus DNA as a probe labelled with ^{32}P by the nick translation procedure. Viral DNA was found to be integrated into cellular DNA in both liver tumour and liver non-tumour tissue in patients with hepatocellular carcinoma as demonstrated by hybridisation of high-molecular-weight DNA after digestion with Hind III and Eco R1 endonucleases. Integrated viral DNA was also found in patients with cirrhosis with or without chronic active hepatitis. Free hepatitis B virus DNA was found in the liver in two patients with chronic persistent hepatitis and in one patient with chronic active hepatitis. Restriction endonuclease patterns in two patients with acute hepatitis B strongly suggested viral DNA integration. If these findings are confirmed by the examination of a large number of patients with acute hepatitis B, then viral integration seems to occur early in the course of infection.

Viral integration is a critical event in cell transformation by some viruses. The long terminal repeat (LTR) sequences of retroviruses, when integrated at appropriate cellular DNA sites, appear to influence directly the expression of cellular oncogenes resulting in cell transformation – the 'promoter-insertion' mechanism. The observations reported so far are not consistent with such a promoter-insertion mechanisms. However, integration at cellular DNA sites adjacent to new and as yet undescribed cellular oncogenes would not be detected by hybridisation with known oncogene probes.

Infection of cells with retroviruses and other viruses can result in point mutations, translocations or other rearrangements of cellular DNA. Such virus effects on cellular DNA could alter the structure or expression of cellular oncogenes, resulting in cell transformation without an apparent lasting viral DNA insert – a 'hit and run' mechanism[19] – or with residual viral sequences. The findings described for hepatitis B virus and the phylogenetically related animal hepatitis B viruses are consistent with such a mechanism[20].

Hepatitis B-like Viruses in Animals: the Hepadna Viruses

A number of human hepatitis B-like viruses have been identified recently in lower animals (other than the great apes).

Snyder[21] reported the presence of liver cancer in 22 out of 76 eastern wood-chucks (*Marmota monax*) which lived longer than 4 years in an established colony. In addition, lesions of chronic active hepatitis and sometimes cirrhosis were usually found in the non-tumour tissue. Examination by electron microscopy of sera collected from the captive woodchucks revealed virus particles which resemble closely human hepatitis B virus[22]. Human hepatitis B virus and the woodchuck hepatitis virus share several characteristics. Infection with either virus results in the accumulation in blood of large amounts of excess virus coat protein in the form of spherical and tubular particles measuring 20–25 nm in diameter. Both are 40–45 nm double-shelled or solid particles with a nucleocapsid containing double-stranded circular DNA with a gap, and both contain a viral DNA polymerase. Each virus is associated with chronic hepatitis and hepato-cellular carcinoma. Antigenic cross-reactivity has been reported between the cores of the two viruses, but only minor common antigenic determinants were identified on the virus surface protein. A small region of 100–150 base pairs of nucleic acid homology, measured by liquid hybridisation, was found in the genomes of the two viruses. It seems likely that this 3–5% of nucleic acid homology represents one or two regions of nearly identical nucleotide sequence. The DNA of human hepatitis B virus and the DNA of woodchuck hepatitis virus have been cloned in the vector lambda gtWES. This was then sub-cloned into the kanamycin-resistant plasmid pA01. Comparison of the recombinant DNAs with authentic virus DNAs by specific hybridisation, size and restriction enzyme analysis showed that the recombinants contained the complete genome of each virus. The nucleic acid homology between the two viral DNAs was confirmed with the cloned DNAs. The woodchuck hepatitis virus and the human hepatitis virus are thus phylogenetically related.

Another virus which is related to human hepatitis B has been described in Beechey ground squirrels (*Spermophilus beecheyi*) in Northern California. Common features with the human hepatitis B virus include virus morphology; size and structure of the viral DNA, a virion DNA polymerase which repairs a single-stranded region in the double-stranded circular genome; cross-reacting surface viral antigens; antigen–antibody systems similar to hepatitis B *e* antigen and the core antigen; and persistent infection, with viral antigen present continuously in the blood. The antigenic and structural relationships between the surface antigens of the human hepatitis B virus, the ground squirrel hepatitis B virus and the woodchuck hepatitis virus have been described in detail[20].

The differences in pathogenicity of these three viruses are notable. While persistent infection in infected ground squirrels is common in endemic areas and the titre of the virus, as measured by viral DNA polymerase activity, is high, there is little or no evidence of hepatitis in infected ground squirrels. In persistently infected squirrels followed up in the laboratory for over 2 years, only the mildest form of inflammation of the liver was found in some animals, and none of 25 ground squirrels developed cirrhosis or liver cancer. The complete DNA sequence of the ground squirrel hepatitis virus has not yet been published, but cross-hybridisation studies show a significant degree of homology between the DNA of human hepatitis B virus and the ground squirrel hepatitis virus. The findings so far indicate that the coding sequences for the major surface antigen polypeptide and the major core polypeptide coding sequence of the three mammalian hepatitis viruses have homologous regions with similar locations in relation to the unique physical features of the DNA of the virions.

The fourth member of this group of viruses was discovered in some domesticated ducks (*Anas domesticus*) in the People's Republic of China following the observation of frequent liver cancer in Pekin ducks. Approximately 10% of Pekin ducks in some commercial flocks in the USA carry a hepatitis B-like virus, named duck hepatitis B virus. This species of duck was originally imported from China in the nineteenth century. The duck hepatitis B virus is similar morphologically to the three mammalian viruses, although the spherical particles are larger and more pleomorphic, and tubular forms have not been found.

The viral genome is circular and partially single-stranded, and an endogenous DNA polymerase can convert the DNA genome to a complete double-stranded circular form with a size of approximately 3000 base pairs. Examination for viral DNA in the organs of infected birds revealed preferential localisation in the liver. The virus is transmitted vertically, and infected ducklings may develop persistent viraemia. Studies on antigenic analysis and nucleotide sequences are in progress.

In summary, therefore, various studies, including comparative pathology and comparative virology of infected eastern woodchucks and Pekin ducks and the mode of replication of the hepadna viruses, have clearly demonstrated that there is a strong and specific association between persistent hepatitis B infection and hepatocellular carcinoma, and it is likely that this association is causal in up to 80% of such cancers in man[1]. However, factors other than hepatitis B virus may be implicated. It is possible that hepatocellular carcinoma is the cumulative result of several cofactors or hepatocarcinogens (including genetic, immunological, nutritional and hormonal factors), mycotoxins (particularly aflatoxin), chemical carcinogens and other environmental influences (including alcohol), and that hepatitis B virus acts either as a carcinogen or as a cocarcinogen in persistently infected hepatocytes (see References 23, 24 for review).

Nevertheless, the evidence of the association between the carrier state of hepatitis B and hepatocellular carcinoma in the majority of patients is such that active immunisation with hepatitis B vaccines is being evaluated in field trials in several countries as a means of preventing infection and long-term risk of developing primary liver cancer. Development of 'preventive measures specific to cancers that are preventable in the countries concerned, leading to a significant reduction in the incidence of these cancers' is one of the three main targets of the WHO Cancer Control Programme. The evidence summarised above demonstrates that the scientific knowledge accumulated to date in the case of hepatitis B and hepatocellular carcinoma now allows such measures to be taken by active immunisation using the currently licensed plasma-derived hepatitis B vaccines (Fig. 4.2). Rapid progress is also being made with the sub-unit polypeptide vaccines (Fig. 4.3), vaccines prepared by recombinant DNA techniques, and with chemically synthesised vaccines (Fig. 4.4).

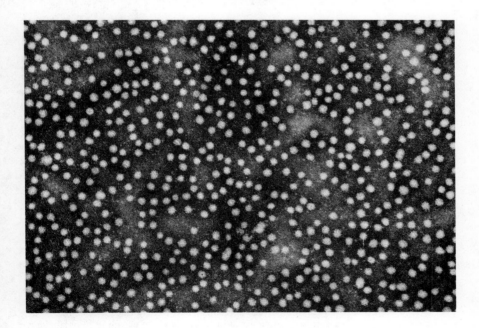

Fig. 4.2   Electron micrograph of hepatitis B vaccine purified from serum. The preparation consists exclusively of small spherical surface antigen particles. × 252 000

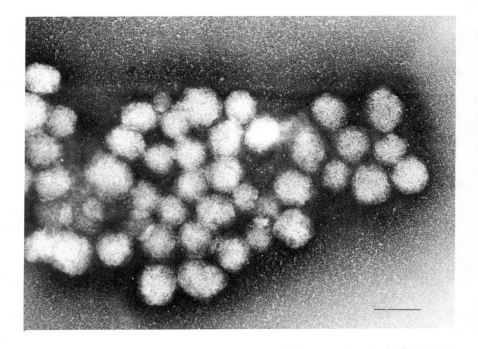

Fig. 4.3   Electron micrograph of hepatitis B surface antigen polypeptides aggregated in the form of micelles. The micelles consist of two polypeptides: the major antigenic component, polypeptide 1, with a molecular weight of 23 000, and its glycosylated form, with a molecular weight of 28 000. Bar = 200 nm

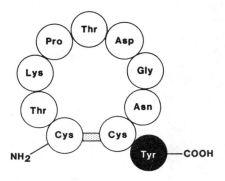

Fig. 4.4   A sequence of hepatitis B surface antigen, 137 to 149, synthesised chemically by a solid-phase technique. A tyrosine residue has been added (Tyr) to permit of radiolabelling, and the sequence is in the cyclical form produced by the introduction of a disulphide bond between the two cysteine residues. (For details see Reference 28 and Brown SE et al. (1984), *Journal of Immunological Methods*, 72: 41–48)

Prevention of the Carrier State of Hepatitis B Virus and of Liver Cancer by Immunisation

Passive Immunisation

Passive immunisation against hepatitis B by the administration of hepatitis B immunoglobulin has been available for nearly a decade, and it has been used with substantial effectiveness for post-exposure prophylaxis within 48 h after exposure after a single acute accidental inoculation and for interrupting maternal-to-infant transmission. The results of small non-randomised studies, and more recently controlled studies, have shown that it is possible to prevent perinatal transmission of hepatitis B virus from surface antigen and *e* antigen carrier mothers to 70–80% of infants by the administration of hepatitis B immuno-globulin at birth, repeated at varying intervals thereafter. However, infection still occurs in many instances (range 20–40%), and later as a result of horizontal transmission for contacts. The importance of administering the first dose of immunoglobulin within a few hours of birth has been emphasised[25].

Active Immunisation

The production of hepatitis B vaccine from the excess surface antigen protein coat of the virus collected from the plasma of asymptomatic carriers is an ingenious, though highly unusual, solution to the repeated failure to grow the virus in tissue culture. The surface antigen is purified by several physical and biological procedures and inactivated. The currently licensed plasma-derived vaccines which meet the WHO Requirements of 1981, revised in 1983, have been shown to be safe and effective, and have not been associated with a risk of transmission of the acquired immune deficiency syndrome or other infectious agent[26]. Vaccines produced by recombinant DNA techniques in eukaryotic cells, particularly yeast, are at a stage of clinical evaluation[27], progress is being made with the development of chemically synthesised hepatitis B peptide vaccines[28], and live recombinant vaccinia virus vaccines are promising[29].

Although the priorities for immunisation against hepatitis B are not the same for each country or geographical region, since the needs are dictated by differing epidemiological patterns, cultural and sexual practices, socioeconomic factors and the environment, it is evident that the prevention of perinatal transmission has the highest priority for children born to mothers in 'high-risk' groups and for susceptible women of childbearing age and their newborn infants in endemic areas. This has been clearly demonstrated by the pioneer studies carried out in Senegal[30] and in Taiwan[31]. The plasma-derived vaccines were highly immunogenic and there was no interference by circulating maternal antibodies. Nevertheless, the protection afforded by the vaccine alone was about 70%, a rate which is similar to the efficacy of passive protection when multiple injections of hepatitis B immunoglobulin are used.

Passive–Active Immunisation

Various temporal combinations of hepatitis B immunoglobulin and hepatitis B vaccine have now been extensively evaluated in Taiwan[31] and in Hong Kong[32], and smaller studies were conducted in Japan, in Holland and elsewhere. A number of trials are still in progress. Analysis of the results of the trials in Taiwan and Hong Kong, which are areas of high endemicity, has shown that combined passive–active prophylaxis improved the protective efficacy in infants born to hepatitis B e antigen carrier mothers to over 90%, whereas in the untreated group development of the carrier state ranged from 73% to 88%.

Although it is difficult to recommend precise immunisation schedules at present, since an international standard preparation of the vaccine is not yet available to permit of direct comparisons between different vaccines, it is clear that combined prophylaxis is the method of choice for protection of infants born to e antigen-positive mothers, and this should be extended to babies born to surface antigen carrier-mothers who are e antibody-negative. Ideally, it has been suggested that infants born to all surface antigen-positive mothers including those with anti-e should be immunised, although it is recognised that the risk of perinatal infection in the latter group is very small. It should be noted, however, that unless these children are actively immunised, they are at a continuing risk of infection by horizontal transmission later in life.

However, the relative scarcity of hepatitis B immunoglobulin and its cost and the current high cost of the licensed hepatitis B vaccines prepared from plasma preclude large-scale prophylaxis at present. Nevertheless, the fact that multiple doses of immunoglobulin as compared with a single dose at birth did not offer significant advantage when combined with a course of vaccine is encouraging. Second, the vaccine is highly immunogenic in infants and the dose could be reduced substantially. Third, vaccines produced by recombinant DNA techniques should prove to be equally effective and substantially cheaper; and there is also the longer-term prospect of cheap chemically synthesised vaccines.

Given sufficient resources, protection by combined immunisation against hepatitis B of all newborn infants at risk is within reach. The principal health benefits will include dramatic reduction of the persistent carrier rate, reduction in morbidity and mortality from chronic liver disease, and prevention of a substantial proportion of hepatocellular carcinomas[33].

Acknowledgements

The hepatitis research programme at the London School of Hygiene and Tropical Medicine is supported by generous grants from the Medical Research Council, the Department of Health and Social Security, the Wellcome Trust, the World Health Organization and Organon B.V. The hepatitis B vaccine development at the London School of Hygiene and Tropical Medicine is generously supported by the British Technology Group (formerly the National Research Development Corporation), the Department of Health and Social Security, the Wellcome Trust and the Commission of the European Economic Community.

References

1. World Health Organization (1983) Prevention of primary liver cancer. Report of a WHO Meeting. World Health Organization Technical Report Series, no 691, Geneva
2. Zuckerman AJ, Sun T-t, Linsell A, Stjernsward J (1983) Prevention of primary liver cancer. Lancet 1: 463–465
3. Sherman M, Shafritz DA (1984) Hepatitis B virus and hepatocellular carcinoma: molecular biology and mechanistic considerations. Seminars in Liver Disease 4: 98–112
4. Beasley RP, Hwang L-Y (1984) Hepatocellular carcinoma and hepatitis B virus. Seminars in Liver Disease 4: 113–121
5. Zuckerman AJ (1974) Viral hepatitis, the B antigen and liver cancer. Cell 1: 65–67
6. Zuckerman, AJ, Dunne A (1974) Hepatitis, hepatocarcinogens and hepatoma. Gazetta Sanitaria 23: 3–11
7. World Health Organization (1977) Advances in viral hepatitis. World Health Organization Technical Report Series, No 602, Geneva
8. Alexander JJ, Bey EM, Geddes EW, Lecatsas G (1976) Establishment of a continuously growing cell line from primary carcinoma of the liver. South African Medical Journal 50: 2124–2128
9. Skelly J, Copeland JA, Howard CR, Zuckerman AJ (1979) Hepatitis B surface antigen produced by a human hepatoma cell line. Nature 282: 617–618
10. Aden DP, Fogel A, Plotkin S, Damjanov I, Knowles BB (1979) Controlled synthesis of HBsAg in a differentiated human liver-carcinoma derived cell line. Nature 282: 615–616
11. Das PK, Nayak NC, Tsiquaye KN, Zuckerman AJ (1980) Establishment of a human hepatoma cell line releasing hepatitis B surface antigen. British Journal of Experimental Pathology 61: 648–654
12. Desmyter J, de Groote J, Ray MB, Bradburne AF, Desmet V, De Somer P, Alexander J (1980) HBsAg-producing human hepatoma cell line: tumours in nude mice and interferon properties. In: Bianchi L, Gerok W, Sinkinger K, Stalder GA (eds) Virus and the liver. MTP, Lancaster, p 217–221
13. Summers J, Mason WS (1982) Replication of the genome of a hepatitis B-like virus by reverse transcription of an RNA intermediate. Cell 29: 403–415
14. Weiser B, Gane D, Seeger C, Varmus HE (1983) Closed circular viral DNA and asymmetrical heterogeneous forms in livers from animals infected with ground squirrel hepatitis virus. Journal of Virology 48: 1–9
15. Fowler MJF, Monjardino J, Tsiquaye KN, Zuckerman AJ, Thomas HC (1984) The mechanism of replication of hepatitis B virus: evidence of asymmetric replication of the two DNA strands. Journal of Medical Virology 13: 83–91
16. Miller RH, Tran C-T, Marion PL, Robinson WS (1984) Replication of hepatitis B virus DNA. In: Viral hepatitis: Proceedings of the 1984 International Symposium. Vyas GN, Dienstag JL, Hoofnagle JH (eds) Greene and Stratton, Orlando, p 629
17. Burrell CJ, Gowans EJ, Jilbert AR, Lake JR, Marmion, BP (1982) Hepatitis B virus DNA detection by in situ cytohybridization: implications for viral replication strategy and pathogenesis of chronic hepatitis. Hepatology 2 (Supplement): 85–91
18. Brechot C, Hadchouel M, Scotto J, Fonck M, Potet F, Vyas GN, Tiollias P (1981) State of hepatitis B virus DNA in hepatocytes of patients with hepatitis B surface antigen-positive and -negative liver diseases. Proceedings of the National Academy of Sciences USA 78: 3906–3910

19. Galloway DA, McDougal JK (1983) The oncogenic potential of herpes simplex viruses: evidence for a 'hit and run' mechanism. Nature 302: 21–24
20. Robinson WS, Marion PL, Miller RH (1984) The Hepadna viruses of animals. Seminars in Liver Disease 4: 347–360
21. Snyder RL (1968) Hepatomas of captive woodchucks. American Journal of Pathology 52: 32
22. Summers J, Smolec MJ, Snyder RL (1978) A virus similar to human hepatitis B virus associated with hepatitis and hepatoma in woodchucks. Proceedings of the National Academy of Sciences USA 75: 4533–4537
23. Zuckerman AJ (1982) Primary hepatocellular carcinoma and hepatitis B virus. Transactions of the Royal Society of Tropical Medicine and Hygiene 76: 711–718
24. Arthur MJP, Hall AJ, Wright R (1984) Hepatitis B, hepatocellular carcinoma and strategies for prevention. Lancet 1: 607–610
25. Beasley RP, Hwang L-Y, Lin C-C, Stevens CE, Wang K-Y, Sun T-S, Hsieh F-J, Szmuness W (1981) Hepatitis B immune globulin (HBIG) efficacy in the interruption of perinatal transmission of hepatitis B carrier state. Lancet 2: 388–393
26. Zuckerman AJ (1984) Who should be immunised against hepatitis B? British Medical Journal 289: 2243–2244
27. McAleer WJ, Buynak EB, Maigetter RZ, Wampler DE, Miller WJ, Hilleman MR (1984) Human hepatitis B vaccine from recombinant yeast. Nature 307: 178–180
28. Brown SE, Howard CR, Zuckerman AJ, Steward MW (1984) Affinity of antibody responses in man to hepatitis B vaccine determined with synthetic peptides. Lancet 2: 184–187
29. Moss B, Smith GL, Gerin JL, Purcell RH (1984) Live recombinant vaccinia virus protects chimpanzees against hepatitis B. Nature 311: 67–69
30. Maupas P, Chiron J-P, Barim F, Coursaget P, Goudeau A, Perrim J, Denir P, Diop Mar I (1981) Efficacy of hepatitis B vaccine in prevention of HBsAg carrier state in children. Controlled trial in an endemic area (Senegal). Lancet 1: 289–292
31. Beasley RP, Hwang L-Y, Lee GC-Y, Lan C-C, Roan C-H, Huang F-Y, Chen C-L (1983) Prevention of perinatally transmitted hepatitis B virus infections with hepatitis B immune globulin and hepatitis B vaccine. Lancet 2: 1099–1102
32. Wong VCW, Ip HMH, Reesink HW, Lelie PN, Reerlink-Brongers EE, Yeung CY, Ma HK (1984) Prevention of the HBsAg carrier state in newborn infants of mothers who are chronic carriers of HBsAg and HBeAg by administration of hepatitis B vaccine and hepatitis B immunoglobulin. Lancet 1: 921–926
33. Zuckerman AJ (1984) Perinatal transmission of hepatitis B. Archives of Diseases in Childhood 59, no 11: 1007–1009

Human Papillomavirus Infections and Prospects for Vaccination

---

Introduction

The infectious aetiology of human warts was established in 1907 by Ciuffo[1], who successfully induced warts in volunteers after injection of cell-free extracts from common warts (verrucae vulgares). Warts occur in man as well as in a wide variety of animals, including Bolivian side-neck turtles[2], African gray parrots[3] and Indian elephants[4], among many other species. It appears that at least the majority of these papillomatous proliferations is caused by papillomaviruses. These viruses are regarded as a sub-group of the genus papovaviruses[5], although they have very little in common with the polyomavirus sub-group. On the basis of structural features, the genomic organisation and biological characteristics, it would be justified to regard the papillomavirus group as an independent genus.

The papillomavirus particle has a diameter of about 55 nm, is composed of 72 capsomeres[6,7] and contains a double-stranded circular DNA of approximately 8 kb[8]. The physical structure of the particle suggests already that it is fairly resistant to chemical and thermal inactivation.

The structure of the papillomavirus DNA has been clarified recently[9-11]. Only one of the two DNA strands is transcribed in one direction. The DNA reveals a number of open reading frames, two of which, L2 and L1, can be assigned to late functions, being responsible for structural viral proteins. Up to eight open reading frames are found in the early region of the viral genome. No intracellular protein has yet been identified originating from any of these reading frames, although active transcription of these regions has been revealed in a number of different systems[11-15]. Thus, an equivalent to T antigens of polyoma-type viruses has not yet been demonstrated in papillomavirus-infected cells.

The rapidly increasing interest in the papillomavirus group in recent years results from their suspected role in common human cancers[16-18] and from the use of papillomavirus DNA as episomal vector systems for mammalian cells[19]. The first aspect, in particular, raises the question as to whether vaccination programmes can be developed for prevention of specific cancers and whether there exists a chance of immunological interference for the treatment of existing papillomas. The data available at present on immunological control of papillomavirus infections are scarce and will be the main subject of this review.

Biology of Papillomavirus Infections

In experimental animals as well as in human volunteers transmission experiments have been carried out and revealed the time period elapsing before papillomatous proliferations became visible. In rabbits infected with Shope papillomavirus an incubation period of 3–8 weeks has been reported[20]. Fibroepitheliomas induced in cattle by bovine papillomavirus type 1 or 2 appear after a latency period of 4–6 weeks[21]. In human infection the latency period varies from several weeks up to several months[1,22]. In human laryngeal papillomatosis, which appears to originate frequently from a perinatal infection with genital papillomaviruses[23-25], clinical symptoms are often not apparent before one or more years.

Table 5.1 lists some of the proliferative conditions in man which are associated with and most likely caused by papillomavirus infections. The list is certainly incomplete, since at least flat cervical lesions[26,27] and oral leukoplakias[28] would have to be included after a more careful analysis of the associated papillomavirus types.

Table 5.1   Benign tumours associated with and probably induced by papillomaviruses

Tumour	Localisation	HPV types
Verruca vulgaris (common wart)	Preferentially extremities, trunk	HPV 1, 2, 4, 7
Verruca plana (flat wart)	Face, extremities, trunk	HPV 3, 10, 29
Condyloma acuminatum (genital wart)	External and internal genital sites	HPV 6, 11
Laryngeal papilloma	Vocal cord	HPV 11, 6
Focal epithelial hyperplasia Heck	Oral mucosa	HPV 13, 1
Genital Bowen's disease and Bowenoid papulosis	External genital sites	HPV 16, 18
Epidermodysplasia verruciformis	Generalised verrucosis	HPV 3, 5, 8–10, 12, 14, 15, 17, 19–25, 26, 29

Although the majority of lesions listed in Table 5.1 are typical papillomas, Bowen's disease and Bowenoid papulosis represent remarkable exceptions. Since in vitro experiments have shown that even non-epithelial tissues can be infected by human papillomaviruses (Takada and zur Hausen, unpublished data), the designation 'papilloma' virus may be misleading. It remains to be seen whether papillomas represent the prime manifestation of these infections and whether other types of benign tumours (e.g. fibromas and adenomas) may also be caused by this virus group.

The development of a benign tumour infection by papillomaviruses requires the availability of a growing cell, or at least of a cell which is still capable of resuming its mitotic activity. Warts develop in microlesions or along scratches, probably owing to the accessibility of proliferating cells of the basal layer. Similarly, the frequent occurrence of papillomavirus-induced dysplasias of the cervix within the transformation zone appears to result from infection of proliferating cells at the surface of the squamo-columnar junction.

Infection of cells leads to the uptake and nuclear persistence of viral DNA as a circular episome[29-31]. Usually the DNA persists in a high copy number, ranging between 20 and 800 genome equivalents per cell[32,33], which suggests an initial accumulation of replicated viral DNA within the infected cell. No structural viral proteins, and consequently no viral particle synthesis, takes place within the infected proliferating cell layer. It appears that growing cells actively suppress late functions of the viral genome.

Early functions of the persisting viral DNA are probably responsible for a growth stimulation of the infected cells resulting in increased proliferation and the appearance of a typical papilloma. Depending on the infecting papillomavirus type, most infected tissues retain to some extent their differentiation pattern. As soon as the cells enter the stratum spinosum and lose their proliferative potential, the block for independent viral DNA replication appears to be released. In certain infections some cells immediately on top of the basal cell layer may reveal independent viral DNA replication[34,35]. Upon further differentiation an increasing number of cells reveals evidence for viral DNA replication, in some instances without concomitant production of structural viral proteins. Structural protein synthesis and particle maturation occur in the stratum granulosum and the stratum corneum. Infection with specific papillomavirus types may lead to the production of large quantities of viral particles, permitting of the isolation of milligram amounts of viral particles from individual papillomas.

The peculiar restriction of particle maturation to highly differentiated cells may represent the prime reason for our present inability to propagate papillomaviruses in tissue culture systems (see reviews in References 36 and 37). Up to now it appears to be impossible to simulate the exact conditions of in vivo differentiation. Thus, all in vitro studies on papillomaviruses depend on isolation of viral components from biopsy material, on molecular cloning of viral DNA and on the expression of the latter in artificial systems.

Plurality of Papillomavirus Types

In recent years the plurality of papillomavirus types has become apparent[38-40].

To date, more than 30 individual types of human papillomaviruses (HPVs) have been characterised. Typing depends entirely on the relatedness of cloned HPV DNA to established prototypes[41]. Table 5.1 lists the identified HPV types and their association with benign tumours.

There exists a remarkable site specificity of HPV and animal papillomavirus types. HPV 1, for instance, is preferentially found in plantar warts and HPV 2 in hand warts[40]; HPV 6, 11, 16 and 18 are typical genital isolates[17,18,24,42]; and HPV 13 obviously prevails in the oral mucosa[43]. A virus causing laryngeal papillomatosis in dogs represents a notable example of the site specificity of papillomavirus types. Cell-free extracts of such laryngeal papillomas induce papillomas only if inoculated into the vocal cord of other dogs but not when inoculated in the oral mucosa (Olson, personal communication). This points to a remarkable target cell specificity of papillomavirus infections and suggests a long adaptation period of individual types to specifically differentiated tissues.

The target cell specificity of HPVs and animal papillomaviruses probably also accounts for the regular failures of interspecies transmission of these agents. Only fibroepithelioma viruses of cattle and deer appear to represent an exception. They transform rodent cells in tissue culture[44,45] and induce fibromas, fibrosarcomas, sarcoids, meningiomas or chondromas, depending on the route of inoculation[30,44,46-48]. The equine sarcoids apparently result from natural transmission of bovine papillomaviruses[30,31]. A human papillomavirus type, HPV 7, has been regularly isolated from butchers only[49,50]. It appears to be present in warts of butchers all over the world and has only once been isolated from a wart of long duration derived from a patient who has never been a meat handler (de Villiers et al., unpublished data). This 'profession-specific' infection may suggest another example of interspecies transmission, although a corresponding agent has not yet been identified in animals.

The macroscopic difference between papillomas induced by different types of papillomaviruses is paralleled by the histological appearance of the respective proliferations[49,51-53]. The cytopathogenic changes induced by individual types of HPVs differ substantially and may provide a first clue to the agent responsible for the respective lesion. The most typical change induced by several types of papillomaviruses is the 'koilocyte'[54], representing a cell with a pycnotic nucleus and a vacuolated cytoplasm which results in the typical 'owl-eye'-like appearance. The identification of koilocytotic cells in cervical dysplasias provided the first hint of a papillomavirus aetiology of these lesions[26]. However, there exist papillomavirus infections without accompanying koilocytotic changes.

Epidemiology of HPV Infections

Production and release of HPV particles within the stratum granulosum and the stratum corneum as well as the physical stability of the viral particles guarantee the successful survival of those infections. The virus appears to require the presence of microlesions in order to reach susceptible target cells.

One other aspect governing the epidemiology of HPV infections is the long persistence of warts, ranging from several months to more than two decades, with apparently continuous virus production at the surface of the lesion. In addition, viral genomes may even persist after regression of a papilloma and may lead to recurrences under conditions of hormonal stimulation or immuno-suppression (reviewed in Reference 37).

Individual HPV types have been found in every human population which has been carefully investigated. A wide variety of virus types has been described in epidermodysplasia verruciformis patients[55]. Although this is an extremely rare condition, it is found in virtually all populations all over the world. The same types are present in Asian, African, American and European patients[56-62]. This is a clear-cut indication that the respective virus types must be present in the general population, although the lesions they induce in healthy individuals should be rather inconspicuous and probably escape detection in most cases.

Sub-types of HPV 6 found in the German population[63] are also found in Japan (Kawana et al., personal communication). This, again, suggests a remarkable genetic stability of the various HPV types and sub-types, and stresses the successful survival of members of this virus group.

The age incidence of papillomavirus infections depends on the infecting virus type. Verrucae planae and verrucae vulgares prevail in younger age groups, whereas condylomata acuminata and genital Bowenoid papulosis closely follow the age distribution of venereal diseases[23,64]. It is very likely that the latter conditions are almost exclusively transmitted by sexual contacts.

Particularly interesting is the age distribution of laryngeal papillomas. As outlined before, young children are preferentially infected, which points to a perinatal period of infection. HPV 11 and 6, both viruses found in condylomata acuminata, are regularly present in laryngeal papillomas. Thus, it appears that the vocal cord is particularly susceptible to genital papillomavirus infections. Since iatrogenic dissemination into the trachea has been recorded frequently (reviewed in Reference 37), tracheal epithelia should also be susceptible to these infections.

Other papillomavirus infections of the mucosa have barely been investigated up to now. Apart from the focal epithelial hyperplasia (Heck) and oral leuko-plakias[28,65], little attention has as yet been paid to these localisations.

However, the occasional presence of HPV DNA in carcinomas of the lung[66], the larynx (Kahn et al., unpublished data: Stremlau et al., unpublished data) and the oral cavity[28] points to a pathognomonic significance of these infections.

Malignant Conversion of Papillomavirus-induced Tumours

The Shope papillomavirus (cottontail-rabbit papillomavirus, CRPV) was the first DNA-containing virus shown to regularly induce papillomas in domestic rabbits which at high frequency subsequently converted into carcinomas[67-69]. The carcinomas metastasised and eventually killed the animals. Although malignant conversion also occurs in the papillomavirus' natural host, the cottontail rabbit, spontaneous regression of the papillomas is much more frequent in the latter species. In domestic rabbit malignant conversion is most frequently observed about 9 months after papilloma induction.

Early studies conducted by Rous and his associates[70-72] noted a co-operative or synergistic interaction between CRPV infection and chemical carcinogens. Tar or methylcholanthrene applied either on papillomas or simultaneously on the virus-inoculated skin significantly enhanced the rate of papillomas converting into carcinomas. Moreover, repeated tarring of the skin, subsequently followed by intravenous inoculation of the virus, resulted in high yields of papillomas and carcinomas.

Additional tumours in cattle and sheep were described in recent years where papillomavirus infection leads to the development of papillomas which upon exposure to physical and chemical carcinogens convert into carcinomas: this is particularly interesting in ocular carcinomas of Hereford cattle, which occur in the unpigmented periphery of the eye in regions of high solar exposure[73]. The precursor lesions of these tumours are typical papillomas and contain papillomavirus particles[74]. Similar lesions occur in sheep around the muzzle and on tips of the ears[75]. In areas of high solar exposure again, these papillomas convert into squamous cell carcinomas.

Jarrett and co-workers[76,77] described alimentary tract papillomas apparently caused by bovine papillomavirus (BPV) type 4. Progression of papillomas to carcinomas occurs in regions where cattle graze on bracken fern, which is known to contain carcinogenic and immunosuppressive substances.

Thus, it appears that in animal systems carcinogenesis induced by specific types of papillomaviruses depends in addition on exposure to physical or chemical carcinogens.

Besides these animal models there exist also some human papillomavirus infections which reveal a high risk for subsequent malignant conversion: epidermodysplasia verruciformis has been mentioned above. This rare condition, characterised by a generalised verrucosis, reveals a high risk for malignant conversion of individual warts at light-exposed sites[22]. Despite the isolation of numerous papillomavirus types from patients with epidermodysplasia verruciformis[58-60], only papillomas containing HPV 5 or HPV 8 and in exceptional cases a few other types also convert into malignant tumours. Here, again, infections with specific types interact with physical carcinogens. It is interesting to note that epidermodysplasia verruciformis is also found in Africans. However, the pigmented skin appears to provide some protection against carcinoma development (see review in Reference 37). Malignant conversion has been observed only rarely in these patients.

The suspicion that human genital cancer is related to papillomavirus infections [16,77a] was recently substantiated by the isolation of HPV 16 and HPV 18 from cancer biopsy material of about 70% of cervical, penile and vulval carcinomas[17,18].

Moreover, the majority of additional cervical carcinomas contain sequences cross-hybridising with HPV DNA under conditions of low stringency, which suggests the presence of related, yet not identified, types of HPV. The regular association of HPV 16 and HPV 18 infections with malignant tumours, their presence in clearly premalignant lesions, such as Bowen's disease, Bowenoid papulosis and advanced cervical intraepithelial neoplasias (CIN), and their absence from typical genital warts support a specific role of these agents in human genital cancer.

This interpretation is underlined by results obtained from tissue culture lines isolated from cervical cancer biopsies. Analysis of HeLa, C4/1 and W 756 cells revealed the presence of HPV 18 DNA[18,78]. The DNA persists in an integrated state and (with the exception of C4/1 cells) is present in multiple copies. In all three lines, as well as in a few tumour biopsies containing HPV 16 DNA, the viral DNA is actively transcribed[78]. It is interesting to note that within these three lines, as well as within a few additional tumour biopsies analysed, the viral DNA integrates close to the $3'$ end of the E_1 or at the $5'$ end of the E_2 open reading frames, which points to a specificity of the integrative events. At present it is not known whether there exist any specific host cell DNA integration sites as well. Since Bowenoid lesions appear to contain HPV 16 DNA as circular episomes[79], the remarkable difference in the state of viral DNA in carcinomas seems to stress a specific role of these virus infections in the development of malignant tumours.

In view of the co-operative or synergistic effect of specific papillomavirus infections with physical or chemical carcinogens in animals and in epidermo-dysplasia verruciformis in man, search for carcinogenic cofactors in human genital cancer seems to be justified. Indeed, heavy and prolonged smoking has been identified as a significant risk factor in cervical cancer[80-84]. Herpes simplex virus infections which share properties with chemical and physical carcinogens[85], in that they are mutagenic[86] and induce selective DNA amplification[87], have been suspected of playing, in addition to smoking, a similar role[88]. It is possible that further, not yet identified, carcinogenic events contribute to the development of cervical cancer. Bacterial and/or protozoal metabolities, for instance, could represent additional cofactors. They could explain the approximately twentyfold higher incidence in cervical cancer when compared with penile and vulval cancer, although HPV infections should be at least as common at penile sites as they are at the cervix.

Laryngeal papillomas, similarly to genital condylomata acuminata, very rarely convert into malignant tumours (see review in Reference 37). Both types of tumour appear to be caused by the same viruses, HPV 6 and HPV11[24,25,42,89]. However, X-irradiation of laryngeal papilkomas for therapeutic reasons resulted in a rather frequent conversion of these tumours into squamous cell carcinomas after latency periods of 5–40 years (see review in Reference 37). This suggests that even HPV infections with a low risk for malignant conversion may lead to carcinoma development after exposure to potent physical carcinogens.

Since carcinoma development of the oropharynx, the larynx and the lung is significantly influenced by carcinogenic habits (e.g. smoking, chewing of betel nut leaves), it is tempting to speculate that these tumours may, in addition, require a specific papillomavirus infection. Indeed, the first HPV-positive carcinomas of the oropharynx[28], the larynx (Kahn et al., to be published; Stremlau et al., to be published) and the lung[66] have already been found. It will be interesting to see whether the isolation of new HPV types present in the mucosa of the respiratory tract results in a significant association of HPV infections with these carcinomas.

State of Viral DNA in Benign and Malignant Tumours

In all benign lesions induced by papillomaviruses the viral DNA persists in an episomal state[29-31]. In carcinomas the situation is more complex. The most detailed data at present available are from human genital cancer[78,79], and have been outlined before. The apparent mode of specific integration of HPV 18 and HPV 16 DNA within their E_2-E_1 open reading frames is of special interest.

The analysis of other carcinomas for integrated papillomavirus DNA has so far been less detailed. Although high-molecular-weight DNA has been observed in small quantities in carcinomas from epidermodysplasia verruciformis patients [61,65], the available data are more compatible with concatameric forms than with integrated HPV DNA.

However, in CRPV-induced rabbit carcinomas and cell lines derived from such tumours there exists clear-cut evidence for CRPV DNA integration[90-94]. The specificity of the integration sites has yet to be assessed.

The available data from genital cancer permit the following speculation: infection with papillomaviruses revealing a high risk for malignant conversion leads to benign lesions of long duration with persisting episomal papillomavirus DNA. Exposure of the persistently infected cells to initiating events leads to high numbers of recombinations between the host cell DNA and episomal viral sequences. From cells in which the viral DNA is specifically opened within the E_2-E_1 open reading frames and inserted into possibly specific domains of host cell DNA, malignant clones arise.

It appears to be likely that, in addition to the described sequence of events, structural rearrangements of persisting episomal viral DNA may also lead to the same consequences.

Papillomavirus-specific Antigens

The papillomavirus genome codes for two structural proteins[9-11]. In view of the problems in propagating papillomaviruses in tissue culture, the proteins are poorly characterised and the kinetics of their synthesis are virtually unknown.

Some studies have been conducted to characterise structural proteins of HPV 1, CRPV, BPV 1 and BPV 2[95-97].

The structural proteins of papillomaviruses reveal, besides type-specific determinants, group-specific antigenicity[98-100]. Antibodies to these antigens have been successfully used to study a wide variety of biopsy materials for papillomavirus particle production[101-103]. It appears that the group-specific determinants are not exposed at the surface of the particles. Therefore, neutralisation of papillomaviruses is probably not achieved by group-specific antisera.

The early functions of papillomavirus genomes are even less well characterised. No antigen has yet been found which corresponds to the T antigens of SV 40 and polyomaviruses, although a stretch of structural homology has been noted between large T of SV 40 and polyomavirus and the putative E_1 protein of papillomaviruses[104]. Since none of the open reading frames of the early region has yet been successfully translated in vitro, a functional assignment is at present impossible.

However, the active transcription of the early region, under conditions of virus latency, strongly suggests the biological importance of this region[12-14,78]. Data obtained from transfection experiments with BPV 1 indicate the existence of two transforming genes in the early region[105]. They may transform independently of each other, although there appears to exist a synergistic interaction. One of the regions, covering E_6 and E_7, is the only early part of HPV 18 and HPV 16 DNA expressed in cervical cancer cell lines and tumour biopsies, whereas the second one, E_2, is either deleted or functionally inactive[78].

Humoral Immune Response to Papillomavirus Antigens

Early data on immunoreactivity against papillomavirus antigens were obtained with pooled preparations of particles from human or animal papillomas. In view of the plurality of papillomavirus types, these studies require reinvestigation.

Almeida and her co-workers[106,107] demonstrated electron microscopically the agglutination of HPV particles by sera obtained from wart carriers. Such studies provided evidence that many wart carriers do not develop measurable titres of antibodies or do so several months after onset of the proliferations[108,109].

By use of a solid-phase radioimmunoassay, HPV 1 antibody production was determined in a random population[110]. Depending on the age group, between 35% and 50% of the sera revealed antibody titres. These titres were usually low, and reached their maximum value at about 20 years of age.

Antibody production against infections with HPV 2, HPV 3, HPV 5 and HPV 8 was also shown by immunodiffusion, immunofluorescence or immune electron microscopy[51,56,111,112]. Similarly, in butchers about 50% revealed antibodies to HPV 7, whereas the majority of controls were negative[51].

According to the available data, antibody titres to papillomavirus antigens appear to be generally low. They increase gradually in the course of the disease[113].

IgM antibodies are initially detectable and apparently persist for prolonged periods of time[114,115]. IgG antibodies are frequently demonstrated shortly before or at the onset of regression of warts[116-119].

The role of humoral immunity in wart regression remains questionable. At least in some patients with persisting warts, significant titres of antibodies directed against the respective virus type have been noted[112].

Cell-mediated Immune Response

There exist some indirect arguments to support the important role of cellular immune responses in the control of wart virus infections. Patients under prolonged immunosuppressive treatment — for instance, kidney and heart transplant recipients — frequently exhibit persisting and disseminated warts[120-122]. Similarly, malignant conditions leading to immunosuppression, particularly Hodgkin's disease and chronic lymphatic leukaemia, frequently reveal pronounced papillomavirus infections[123-126]. More direct evidence for a role of cell-mediated immune mechanisms in papilloma regression originates from studies on wart regression in CRPV-infected rabbits[127-129]. Regressing papillomas reveal mononuclear cell infiltrates which are specifically concentrated in the basal cell layer. In addition, colony inhibition tests pointed to activated cell-mediated functions. Impairment of the immune system by methylprednisolone did not influence latency period, papilloma growth rate, production of virus particles or malignant conversion[130]. It did, however, lead to secondary papillomas and affected significantly the regression rate. Forty-seven per cent of the control animals revealed regressions, whereas 2.5% of the steroid-treated animals showed signs of regression.

In human infections epidermodysplasia verruciformis patients provide evidence for a role forcell-mediated immunity in wart control. These patients frequently reveal impairments in the index of 1-nitro-2,4-dichlorobenzene sensitisation, in E-rosette formation, in lymphocyte transformation and in lymphocyte migration inhibition[131-135], whereas virus-type specific humoral immune functions are well preserved[51]. Other patients with warts of long persistence frequently were less responsive in lymphocyte transformation tests[124] and exhibited fewer T cells[136].

The data suggest that epidermodysplasia verruciformis patients are specifically characterised by impaired cellular immune functions directed against papillomaviruses, which predisposes these patients to these kinds of infections.

In human warts spontaneous regression is accompanied by lymphatic infiltrates, affecting, in particular, the basal cell layer[137], and by the presence of macrophages[138,139]. Although in regressing plantar and common warts no cellular infiltrates were noted in some studies[114,140], obvious signs of inflammation were described in others[141,142]. Thus, available evidence underlines the role of cellular immune functions in wart regression and provides little support for a significant role for humoral responses.

Prospects for Vaccination against HPV Infections

Vaccination against human papillomavirus infections would depend on at least two preconditions: first, that the infections represent a severe medical problem, and second, that infections can be controlled by immune mechanisms.

There exists little doubt today that various infections by papillomaviruses may lead to serious medical problems. In particular, laryngeal papillomatosis in children may result in a life-threatening condition. Similarly, genital warts, which are frequently difficult to remove surgically, may pose serious problems. The association of papillomavirus infections with cervical dysplasia and genital cancer appears to be the most significant condition for consideration of vaccine development. Among females cervical cancer is one of the most frequent malignancies in Africa, South America and South Asia[143]. Even in European countries and in North America it is still an important tumour which deserves special interest. Penile and vulval cancer are less frequent, although some countries such as Uganda and Thailand show a high incidence of penile cancer[143].

Previous consideration of the role of immune functions points to a significant role for cell-mediated immune mechanisms in the control of wart virus infections. Therefore, successful stimulation of these functions could be beneficial in two respects: it could lead to prevention of these infections but at the same time may have therapeutic significance.

The inability to propagate papillomaviruses in tissue culture makes it difficult to obtain sufficient quantities of viral antigens for immunisation by using biopsy materials. This is even more unlikely in genital papillomavirus infections, which are usually characterised by very low yields of viral particles and viral antigens [42,107]. Thus, a conventional approach for the preparation of immunogenic proteins of these viruses appears to be highly unlikely until now.

Today the sequences of HPV 1[10], HPV 6[11], HPV 8 (Pfister et al., unpublished data), HPV 11 (Dartmann et al., to be published) and HPV 16[144] have been determined. In addition, the DNA of all other known papillomavirus genotypes has been cloned and is available in larger quantities. Since all genomes characterised thus far reveal a similar gene organisation, various strategies for vaccine development can be considered:

1. Production of viral antigens in bacterial or eukaryotic cells after cloning the respective genes into suitable expression vectors.

2. Production of synthetic vaccines by synthesis of oligopeptides representing antigenic determinants of papillomavirus proteins.

3. Cloning of specific papillomavirus sequences into other viral DNA (preferentially vaccinia virus) and induction of specific immune responses.

The first two approaches clearly present a problem: it is unlikely that cellular immune functions will be significantly stimulated by inoculating these preparations. The third approach may have a better chance of resulting in a specific stimulation of cell-mediated immune functions.

One other problem concerns the selection of the 'right' gene function for vaccination studies. Late viral genes appear to be expressed exclusively in the stratum granulosum and the stratum corneum, but not in the proliferating cells of the basal cell layer. Antibodies to these proteins may neutralise the virus particles, but it is unlikely that an immune response to viral structural antigens will result in inhibition of growth of papillomavirus-transformed cells. Therefore, it seems to be more appropriate to select early gene functions in order to affect proliferating cells for preventative as well as for therapeutic reasons. Although virtually nothing is known about the expression of these putative proteins in infected cells, the data on spontaneous and systemic wart regression suggest that such proteins are produced and should even be recognisable at the surface of the infected cells. The difficulties in demonstrating early proteins within these cells may result from small quantity or rapid turnover rate. This could lead to the speculation that their low concentration, particularly at the cell membrane, in most instances will not suffice for immunogenic stimulation. If this assumption is correct, vaccines stimulating an immune response against the responsible antigen would, indeed, besides preventative properties, possess therapeutic value.

Thus, the concentration of effort on the generation of such vaccines appears to be justified. One inherent problem will be the exclusion of potentially malignant functions, particularly when functional genes are cloned in viral vector systems.

There exist a number of preliminary hints that specific types of papillomaviruses may be involved in other wide-spread malignant tumours of man, such as lung cancer, laryngeal cancer, oropharyngeal cancer and oesophageal cancer[37,85,145]. It is likely that we have not yet isolated the majority of potentially malignant papillomavirus genotypes in man. Their sequencing and the identification of cross-reacting antigenic determinants seem to be an important prerequisite for vaccine development.

It is anticipated that vaccination will play an important role not only in the prevention of papillomavirus infections, but also in the therapy of these proliferations. It is evident, however, that this field is in the very early phase of its development.

References

1. Ciuffo G (1907) Innesto positivo con filtrado di verrucae volgare. Giorn Ital Mal Venereol 48:12–17
2. Jacobson ER, Gaskin JM, Clubb S, Calderwood MB (1982) Papilloma-like virus infection in Bolivian side-neck turtles. J Am Vet Med Assoc 181:1325–1328
3. Jacobson ER, Maldinich CR, Clubb S, Sundberg JP, Lancaster WD (1983) Papilloma-like virus infection in an African gray parrot. J Am Vet Med Assoc 183:1307–1308
4. Sundberg JP, Russell WC, Lancaster W (1981) Papillomatosis in Indian elephants. J Am Vet Med Assoc 179:1247–1249
5. Melnick JL, Allison AC, Butel JS, Eckhart W, Eddy BE, Kitt S, Levine AJ, Miles JAR, Pagano JS, Sachs L, Vonka V (1974) Papovaviridae. Intervirology 3:106–120
6. Crawford LV, Crawford EM (1963) A comparative study of polyoma and papilloma viruses. Virology 21:258–263
7. Klug A, Finch JT (1965) Structure of viruses of the papilloma-polyoma type. I. Human wart virus. J Molec Biol 11:403–423
8. Kleinschmidt AU, Kass SJ, Williams RC, Knight CA (1965) Cyclic DNA of Shope papilloma virus. J Molec Biol 13:749–756

9. Chen EY, Howley PM, Levinson AD, Seeburg PH (1982) The primary structure and genetic organization of the bovine papilloma-virus type 1 genome. Nature 299: 529–534

10. Danos O, Katinka M, Yaniv M (1982) Human papillomavirus 1a complete DNA sequence: A novel type of genome organization among papovaviridae. EMBO J 1:231–236

11. Schwarz E, Dürst M, Demankowski C, Lattermann O, Zech R, Wolfsperger E, Suhai S, zur Hausen H (1983) DNA sequence and genome organization of genital human papillomavirus type 6b. EMBO J 2:2341–2348

12. Amtmann E, Sauer G (1982) Bovine papilloma virus transcription: Polyadenylated RNA species and assessment of the direction of transcription. J Virol 43:59–66

13. Heilman CA, Engel L, Lowy DR, Howley PM (1982) Virus-specific transcription in bovine papillomavirus transformed mouse cells. Virology 119:22–34

14. Freese UK, Schulte P, Pfister H (1982) Papilloma virus-induced tumors contain a virus-specific transcript. Virology 117:257–261

15. Lehn H, Ernst T-M, Sauer G (1984) Transcription of episomal papillomavirus DNA in human condylomata acuminata and Buschke–Löwenstein tumors. J Gen Virol 65:2003–2010

16. Zur Hausen H (1976) Condylomata acuminata and human genital cancer. Cancer Res 36:794

17. Dürst M, Gissmann L, Ikenberg H, zur Hausen H (1983) A papillomavirus DNA from a cervical carcinoma and its prevalence in cancer biopsy samples from different geographic regions. Proc Natl Acad Sci USA 80:3812–3815

18. Boshart M, Gissmann L, Ikenberg H, Kleinheinz A, Scheurlen W, zur Hausen H (1984) A new type of papillomavirus DNA, its presence in genital cancer biopsies and in cell lines derived from cervical cancer. EMBO J 3:1151–1157

19. Sarver N, Gruss P, Law M-F, Khoury G, Howley PM (1981) Bovine papilloma virus deoxyribonucleic acid: A novel eucaryotic cloning vector. Molec Cell Biol 1:486–496

20. Ito Y (1975) Papilloma-myxoma viruses. In: Becker FF (ed) Cancer: A comprehensive treatise. Plenum, New York, vol 2, p 323–341

21. Olson C, Gordon DE, Robl MG, Lee KP (1969) Oncogenicity of bovine papilloma virus. Arch Environ Health 19:827–837

22. Jablonska S, Dabrowski J, Jakubowicz K (1972) Epidermodysplasia verruciformis as a model in studies on the role of papovaviruses in oncogenesis. Cancer Res 32:583–589

23. Zur Hausen H, Gissmann L, Steiner W, Dippold W, Dregger I (1975) Human papilloma virus and cancer. Bibl Haematol 43:569–571

24. Gissmann L, Diehl V, Schultz-Coulon H-J, zur Hausen H (1982) Molecular cloning and characterization of human papilloma virus DNA derived from a laryngeal papilloma. J Virol 44:393–400

25. Mounts P, Shah KV, Kashima H (1982) Viral etiology of juvenile- and adult onset squamous papilloma of the larynx. Proc Natl Acad Sci USA 79:5425–5429

26. Meisels A, Fortin R (1976) Condylomatous lesions of the cervix and vagina. I. Cytologic patterns. Acta Cytol 20:505–509

27. Meisels A, Roy M, Fortier M, Morin C, Casas-Cordero M, Shah KV, Turgeon H (1981) Human papilloma virus infection of the cervix: The atypical condyloma. Acta Cytol 25:7–16

28. Löning H, Ikenberg H, Becker J, Gissmann L, Hoepfner I, zur Hausen H (1985) Analysis of oral papillomas, leucoplakias and invasive carcinomas for human papillomavirus DNA. J Invest Dermatol (in press)

29. Stevens JG, Wettstein FO (1979) Multiple copies of Shope viral DNA are present in cells of benign and malignant non-virus producing neoplasms. J Virol 30:891–898

30. Lancaster WD, Theilen GH, Olson C (1979) Hybridization of bovine papillomavirus type 1 and type 2 DNA to DNA from virus-induced hamster tumors and naturally occurring equine tumors. Intervirology 11:227–233

31. Amtmann, E, Müller H, Sauer G (1980) Equine connective tissue tumors contain unintegrated bovine papilloma virus DNA. J Virol 35:962–964

32. Lancaster WD, Olson C, Meinke W (1976) Quantitation of bovine papilloma viral DNA in viral-induced tumors. J Virol 17:824–831

33. Lancaster WD, Olson C, Meinke W (1977) Bovine papilloma virus: Presence of virus-

specific DNA sequences in naturally occurring equine tumors. Proc Natl Acad Sci USA 74:524-538

34. Orth G, Jeanteur P, Croissant O (1971) Evidence for and localization of vegative viral DNA replication by autographic detection of RNA-DNA hybrids in sections of tumors induced by Shope papilloma virus. Proc Natl Acad Sci USA 68:1876-1880

35. Grussendorf EI, zur Hausen H (1979) Localization of viral DNA-replication in sections of human warts by nucleic acid hybridization with complementary RNA of human papilloma virus type 1. Arch Dermatol Res 254:55-63

36. Rowson KEK, Mahy BWJ (1967) Human papova (wart) virus. Bacteriol Rev 31:110-131

37. Zur Hausen H (1977) Human papillomaviruses and their possible role in squamous cell carcinoma. In: Arber W et al. (eds) Current topics in microbiology and immunology. Springer, New York, vol 78, p 1-30

38. Gissmann L, zur Hausen H (1976) Human papilloma virus DNA: Physical mapping and genetic heterogeneity. Proc Natl Acad Sci USA 73:1310-1313

39. Gissmann L, Pfister H, zur Hausen H (1977) Human papilloma viruses (HPV): Characterization of four different isolates. Virology 76:569-580

40. Orth G, Favre M, Croissant O (1977) Characterization of a new type of human papillomavirus that causes skin warts. J Virol 24:108-120

41. Coggin JR, zur Hausen H (1979) Workshop of papillomaviruses and cancer. Cancer Res 39:545-546

42. Gissmann L, zur Hausen H (1980) Partial characterization of viral DNA from human genital warts (Condylomata acuminata). Int J Cancer 25:605-609

43. Pfister H, Gassenmaier A, Nürnberger F, Stüttgen G (1983a) Human papilloma virus 5-DNA in a carcinoma of an epidermodysplasia verruciformis patient infected with various human papillomavirus types. Cancer Res 43:1436-1441

44. Boiron M, Levy JP, Thomas M, Friedman JC, Bernard J (1964) Some properties of bovine papilloma virus. Nature 201:423-424

45. Puget A, Favre M, Orth G (1975) Induction de tumeurs fibroblastiques cutanés ou sous cutaneous chez l'Ochotone afghan (Ochotono rufescens) par l'inoculation du virus papilloma bovin. CR Acad Sci Paris 280.2813-2816

46. Friedman JC, Levy JP, Lasneret J, Thomas M, Boiron M, Bernard J (1963) Induction de fibromes son-cutanés chez le hamster dore par inoculation d'extraits acellulaires de papillomes bovins. CR Acad Sci Paris 257:2328-2331

47. Cheville NF (1966) Studies on connective tissue tumors in the hamster produced by bovine papilloma virus. Cancer Res 26:2334-2339

48. Robl MG, Olson C (1968) Oncogenic action of bovine papilloma virus in hamsters. Cancer Res 28:1596-1604

49. Orth G, Jablonska S, Favre M, Croissant O, Obalek S, Jarzabek-Chorzelska M, Jibard N (1981) Identification of papillomaviruses in butchers' warts. J Invest Dermatol 1:97-102

50. Ostrow RS, Krzyzek R, Pass F, Faras AJ (1981) Identification of a novel human papilloma virus in cutaneous warts of meathandlers. Virology 108:21-27

51. Jablonska S, Orth G, Glinski G, Obalek S, Jarzabek-Chorzelska M, Croissant O, Favre M, Rzesa G (1980) Morphology and immunology of human warts and familial warts. In: Bachmann PA (ed) Leukaemias, lymphomas and papillomas: comparative aspects. Taylor and Francis, London, p 107-131

52. Grussendorf EI (1980) Lichtmikroskopische Untersuchungen an typisierten Viruswarzen (HPV-1 und HPV-4). Arch Dermatol Res 268:141-148

53. Gross G, Pfister H, Hagedorn M, Gissmann L (1982) Correlation between human papillomavirus (HPV) type and histology of warts. J Invest Dermatol 78:160-164

54. Koss LG, Durfee GR (1956) Unusual patterns of squamous epithelium of the uterine cervix: cytologic and pathologic study of koilocytotic atypia. Ann NY Acad Sci 63:1245-1261

55. Orth G, Favre M, Breitburd F, Croissant O, Jablonska S, Obalek S, Jarzabek-Chorzelska M, Rzesa G (1980) Epidermodysplasia verruciformis: A model for the role of papillomaviruses in human cancer. In: Essex M, Todaro G, zur Hausen H (eds) Viruses in naturally occurring cancers. Cold Spring Harbor Laboratory, Cold Spring Harbor, New York, p 259-282

56. Pfister H, Fink B, Thomas C (1981) Extrachromosomal bovine papillomavirus type 1 DNA in hamster fibromas and fibrosarcomas. Virology 115:414–418
57. Yutsudo M, Tanigaki T, Tsumori T, Watanabe S, Hakura A (1982) New human papilloma virus isolated from epidermodysplasia verruciformis lesions. Cancer Res 42:2440–2443
58. Kremsdorf D, Jablonska S, Favre M, Orth G (1982) Biochemical characterization of two types of human papillomaviruses associated with epidermodysplasia verruciformis. J Virol 43:436–477
59. Kremsdorf D, Jablonska S, Favre M, Orth G (1983) Human papillomaviruses associated with epidermodysplasia verruciformis. II Molecular cloning and biochemical characterization of human papillomavirus 3a, 8, 10 and 12 genomes. J Virol 48:340–351
60. Kremsdorf D, Favre M, Jablonska S, Obalek S, Rueda LA, Lutzner MA, Blanchet-Bardon C, van Voorst Vader PC, Orth G (1984) Molecular cloning and characterization of the genomes of nine newly recognized papillomavirus types associated with epidermodysplasia verruciformis. J Virol 52:1013–1018
61. Ostrow RS, Bender M, Niimura M, Seki T, Kawashima M, Pass F, Faras AJ (1982) Human papillomavirus DNA in cutaneous primary and metastasized squamous cell carcinomas from patients with epidermodysplasia verruciformis. Proc Natl Acad Sci USA 79:1634–1638
62. Ostrow RS, Zachow K, Watts S, Bender M, Pass F, Faras A (1983) Characterization of two HPV-3 related papillomaviruses from common warts which are distinct clinically from flat warts or epidermodysplasia verruciformis. J Invest Dermatol 80:436–440
63. de Villiers E-M, Gissmann L, zur Hausen H (1981) Molecular cloning of viral DNA from human genital warts. J Virol 40:932–935
64. Oriel JD (1971) Anal warts and anal coitus. Br J Vener Dis 47:373–376
65. Pfister H, Hettich I, Runne U, Gissmann L, Chilf GN (1983) Characterization of human papillomavirus type 13 from focal epithelial hyperplasia Heck lesions. J Virol 47:363–366
66. Stremlau A, Gissmann L, Ikenberg H, Stark M, Bannasch P, zur Hausen H (1985) Human papillomavirus type 16 related DNA in an anaplastic carcinoma of the lung. Cancer (in press)
67. Rous P, Beard JW (1935) The progression to carcinoma of virus-induced rabbit papilloma (Shope). J Exp Med 62:523–548
68. Kidd JG, Rous P (1940) Cancers deriving from the virus papilloma of wild rabbits under natural conditions. J Exp Med 71:469–485
69. Syverton JT (1952) The pathogenesis of the rabbit papilloma-to-carcinoma sequence. Ann NY Acad Sci 54:1126–1140
70. Rous P, Kidd JG (1938) The carcinogen effect of a papilloma virus on the tarred skin of rabbits. I. Description of the phenomenon. J Exp Med 67:399–422
71. Rous R, Friedwald WF (1944) The effect of chemical carcinogens on virus-induced rabbit carcinomas. J Exp Med 79:511–537
72. Rogers S, Rous P (1951) Joint action of a chemical carcinogen and a neoplastic virus to induce cancer in rabbits. Results of exposing epidermal cells to a carcinogenic hydrocarbon at time of infection with the Shope papilloma virus. J Exp Med 93:459–488
73. Spradbrow PB, Hoffman D (1980) Bovine ocular squamous cell carcinoma. Vet Bull 50:449–459
74. Ford JN, Jennings PA, Spradbrow PB, Francis J (1982) Evidence for papillomaviruses in ocular lesions in cattle. Res Vet Sci 32:257–259
75. Vanselow BA, Spradbrow PB (1982) Papillomaviruses, papillomas and squamous cell carcinomas in sheep. Vet Rec 110:561–562
76. Jarrett WFH, McNeil PE, Grimshaw WTR, Selman IE, McIntyre WIM (1978) High incidence area of cattle cancer with a possible interaction between an environmental carcinogen and a papilloma virus. Nature 274:215–217
77. Jarrett WFH (1980) Bovine papillomaviruses and alimentary malignancy. In: Bachmann PA (ed) Leukaemia, lymphomas and papillomas: comparative aspects. Taylor and Francis, London, p 87–91
77a. Zur Hausen H (1975) Oncogenic herpesviruses. Biophys Biochem Acta 417:25–53
78. Schwarz E, Freese UK, Gissmann L, Mayer W, Roggenbuck B, Stremlau A, zur Hausen H

(1985) Structure and transcription of human papillomavirus sequences in cervical carcinoma cells. Nature (in press)
79. Dürst M, Kleinheinz A, Hotz M, Gissmann L (1985) The physical state of human papillomavirus type 16 DNA in benign and malignant genital tumors (submitted for publication)
80. Winkelstein W Jr (1977) Smoking and cancer of the uterine cervix. Am J Epidemiol 106:257-259
81. Wigle DT (1980) Re: 'Smoking and cancer of the cervix: hypothesis'. Am J Epidemiol 111:125-127
82. Clarke EA, Morgan RW, Newman AM (1982) Smoking as a risk factor in cancer of the cervix: additional evidence from a case-control study. Am J Epidemiol 115:59-66
83. Vonka V, Kanka J, Jelinek J, Subrt I, Sucharek A, Havrankova A, Vachal M, Hirsch I, Domorazkova E, Zavadova H, Richterova V, Naprstkova J, Dvorakova V, Svoboda B (1984). Prospective study on the relationship between cervical neoplasia and herpes simplex type-2 virus. I. Epidemiological characteristics. Int J Cancer 33:49-60
84. Vonka V, Kanka J, Hirsch I, Zavadova H, Krcmar M, Suchankova A, Rezakova D, Broucek, J, Press M, Domorazkova E, Svoboda B, Havrankova A, Jelinek J (1984) Prospective study on the relationship between cervical neoplasia and herpes simplex type-2 virus. Herpes simplex type-2 antibody presence in sera taken at enrolment. Int J Cancer 33:61-66
85. Zur Hausen H (1980) The role of viruses in human tumors. Adv Cancer Res 33:77-107
86. Schlehofer JR, zur Hausen H (1982) Induction of mutations within the host genome by partially inactivated herpes simplex virus type 1. Virology 122:471-475
87. Schlehofer JR, Gissmann L, zur Hausen H (1983) Herpes simplex virus induced amplification of SV40 sequences in transformed Chinese hamster embryo cells. Int J Cancer 32:99-103
88. Zur Hausen H (1982) Human genital cancer: Synergism between two virus infections or synergism between a virus infection and initiating events. Lancet ii:1370-1372
89. Gissmann L, Wolnik L, Ikenberg H, Koldovsky U, Schnürch HG, zur Hausen H (1983) Human papillomavirus types 6 and 11 DNA sequences in genital and laryngeal papillomas and in some cervical cancers. Proc Natl Acad Sci USA 80:560-563
90. Wettstein FO, Stevens JG (1981) Transcription of the viral genome in papillomas and carcinomas induced by the Shope virus. Virology 109:448-451
91. Wettstein FO, Stevens JG (1982) Variable-sized free episomes of Shope papilloma virus DNA are present in all non-virus producing neoplasms and integrated episomes are detected in some. Proc Natl Acad Sci USA 79:790-794
92. Favre M, Jibard N, Orth G (1982) Restriction mapping and physical characterization of the cottontail rabbit papillomavirus genome in transplantable VX2 and VX7 domestic rabbit carcinomas. Virology 119:298-309
93. McVay P, Fretz M, Wettstein F, Stevens J, Ito Y (1982) Integrated Shope virus DNA is present and transcribed in the transplantable rabbit tumor Vx-7. J Gen Virol 60:271-278
94. Georges E, Croissant O, Bonneaud N, Orth G (1984) Physical state and transcription of the cottontail rabbit papillomavirus genome in warts and in transplantable VX2 and VX7 carcinomas of domestic rabbits. J Virol 51:530-538
95. Spira G, Estes MH, Dreesman GR, Butel JS, Rawls WE (1974) Papova virus structural polypeptides: Comparison of human and rabbit papilloma viruses with simian virus. Intervirology 3:220-231
96. Favre M, Breitburd F, Croissant O, Orth G (1975) Structural polypeptides of rabbit, bovine and human papillomavirus. J Virol 15:1239-1247
97. Pfister H, Gissmann L, zur Hausen H (1977) Partial characterization of the proteins of human papilloma viruses. Virology 83:131-137
98. Orth G, Jablonska S, Favre M, Croissant O, Jarzabek-Chorzelska M, Rzesa G (1978) Characterization of two types of human papillomavirus in lesions of epidermodysplasia verruciformis. Proc Natl Acad Sci USA 75:1537-1541
99. Jenson AB, Rosenthal JD, Olson C, Pass F, Lancaster WD, Shah K (1980) Immunologic relatedness of papillomaviruses from different species. J Natl Cancer Inst 64:495-500

100. Shah KH, Lewis MG, Jenson AB, Kurman RJ, Lancaster WD (1980) Papillomavirus and cervical dysplasia. Lancet ii:1190

101. Costa J, Howley PM, Bowling MC, Howard R, Bauer WC (1980) Presence of human papilloma viral antigens in juvenile multiple laryngeal papilloma. Am Soc Clin Pathol 75:194-197

102. Lancaster WD, Jenson AB (1981) Evidence for papillomavirus genus-specific antigens and DNA in laryngeal papilloma. Intervirology 15:204-212

103. Dyson JL, Walker PG, Singer A (1984) Human papillomavirus infection of the uterine cervix: Histological appearances in 28 cases identified by immunohistochemical techniques. J Clin Pathol 150:126-130

104. Clertant P, Seif J (1984) A common function for polyoma virus large-T and papillomavirus E1 proteins? Nature 311:276-279

105. Sarver N, Rabson MG, Yang YC, Byrne JC, Howley PM (1984) Localization and analysis of bovine papillomavirus type 1 transforming functions. J Virol 52:377-388

106. Almeida JD, Goffe AP (1965) Antibody to wart virus in human sera demonstrated by electron microscopy and precipitin tests. Lancet ii:1205-1207

107. Almeida JD, Oriel ID, Stannard LM (1969) Characterization of the virus found in human genital warts. Microbios 3:225-232

108. Cubie HA (1976) Failure to produce warts on human skin grafts on 'nude' mice. J Dermatol 94:659-665

109. Pass F, Maizel JV (1973) Wart-associated antigens. II. Human immunity to viral structural proteins. J Invest Dermatol 60:307-311

110. Pfister H, zur Hausen H (1978) Seroepidemiological studies of human papilloma virus (HPV-1) infections. Int J Cancer 21:161-165

111. Jablonska S, Orth G, Jarzabek-Chorzelska M, Obalek S, Glinski W, Favre M, Croissant O (1979) Epidermodysplasia verruciformis versus disseminated verrucae planae: Is epidermodysplasia verruciformis a generalized infection with wart virus? J Invest Dermatol 72:114-119

112. Pfister H, Huchthausen B, Gross G, zur Hausen H (1979) Seroepidemiological studies of bovine papillomavirus infections. J Natl Cancer Inst 62:1423-1425

113. Pyrhönen S (1972) Human wart antibodies in patients with genital and skin warts. Acta Dermatol Vener (Stockholm) 58:427-432

114. Matthews RS, Shirodaria PV (1973) Study of regressing warts by immunofluorescence. Lancet i:689-691

115. Shirodaria PV, Matthews RS (1975) An immunofluorescence study of warts. Clin Exp Immunol 21:329-338

116. Ogilvie MM (1970) Serological studies with human papova (wart) virus. J Hyg 68:479-483

117. Genner J (1971) Verruca vulgaris. II. Demonstration of a complement fixation reaction. Acta Derm Venereol 51:365-373

118. Pyrhönen S, Penttinen K (1972) Wart virus antibodies and the prognosis of wart disease. Lancet ii:1330-1332

119. Pyrhönen S, Johannson E (1975) Regression of warts. An immunological study. Lancet i:592-596

120. Spencer ES, Anderson HK (1970) Clinically evident, non-terminal infections with herpes virus and the wart virus in immunosuppressed renal allograft recipients. Br Med J 3:251-254

121. Starzl TE, Porter KA, Andres G, Halgrimson CG, Hurwitz R, Giles G, Terasaki PJ, Penn J, Schroter GT, Lilly J, Starkie SJ, Putnam CW (1970) Long-term survival after renal transplantation in humans. Ann Surg 172:437-472

122. Koranda FC, Dehmel EM, Kahn G, Penn I (1974) Cutaneous complications in immunosuppressed renal homograft recipients. J Am Med Assoc 229:419-424

123. Perry TL, Harman L (1974) Warts in diseases with immune defects. Cutis 13:359-362

124. Morison WL (1975) Cell-mediated immune responses in patients with warts. Br J Dermatol 93:553-556

125. Reid TMS, Fraser NG, Kernohan IR (1976) Generalized warts and immune deficiency. Br J Dermatol 95:559-564

126. Ward M, le Roux A, Small WP, Sircus W (1977) Malignant lymphoma and extensive

viral wart formation in a patient with intestinal lymphangiectasia and lymphocyte depletion. Postgrad Med J 53:753-757

127. Kreider JW (1963) Studies on the mechanism responsible for the spontaneous regression of the Shope rabbit papilloma. Cancer Res 23:1593-1599

128. Kreider JW (1980) Neoplastic progression of the Shope rabbit papilloma. Cold Spring Harbor Conf Cell Prolif 7:283-300

129. Hellström I, Evans CA, Hellström KE (1969) Cellular immunity and its serum-mediated inhibition in Shope-virus-induced rabbit papillomatosis. Int J Cancer 4:601-607

130. McMichael H (1967) Inhibition by methylprednisolone of regress of the Shope rabbit papilloma. J Natl Cancer Inst 39:55-65

131. Glinski W, Jablonska S, Langner A, Obalek S, Haftek M, Proniewska M (1976) Cell-mediated immunity in epidermodysplasia verruciformis. Dermatologica 153:218-227

132. Glinski W, Obalek S, Jablonska S, Orth G (1981) T cell defect in patients with epidermodysplasia verruciformis due to human papillomavirus type 3 and 5. Dermatologica 162:141-147

133. Prawer SE, Pass F, Vance JC, Greenberg EJ, Yunis EJ, Zelickson AS (1977) Depressed immune function in epidermodysplasia verruciformis. Arch Dermatol 113:495-499

134. Kienzler JL, Laurent R, Coppey J, Favre M, Orth G, Coupez L, Agache P (1979) Epidermodysplasia verruciforme. Donnes ultra-structurales, virologiques et photo-biologiques; a propos d'une observation. Ann Dermatol Venereol 106:549-563

135. Obalek S, Glinski W, Haftek M, Orth G, Jablonska S (1980) Comparative studies on cell mediated immunity in patients with different warts. Dermatologica 161:73-83

136. Chretien JH, Esswein JG, Garagusi VF (1978) Decreased T cell levels in patients with warts. Arch Dermatol 114:213-215

137. Takigawa M, Tagami H, Watanabe S, Ogino A, Imamura S, Ofugi S (1977) Recovery processes during regression of plane warts. Arch Dermatol 113:1214-1218

138. Oguchi M, Komura J, Tagami H, Ofuji S (1981) Ultrastructural studies of spontaneously regressing plane warts. Langerhans cells show marked activation. Arch Dermatol Res 271:55-61

139. Oguchi M, Komura J, Tagami H, Ofuji S (1981) Ultrastructural studies of spontaneously regressing plane warts. Macrophages attack verruca-epidermal cells. Arch Dermatol Res 270:403-411

140. Brodersen I, Genner J (1973) Histological and immunological observations on common warts in regression. Acta Derm Venereol 53:461-464

141. Berman A, Winkelmann RK (1980) Involuting common warts. Clinical and histopathologic findings. J Am Acad Dermatol 3:356-362

142. Berman A, Domnitz JM, Winkelmann RK (1982) Plantar warts recently turned black. Clinical and histopathologic findings. Arch Dermatol 118:47-51

143. Waterhouse J, Muir C, Shanmugaratnam K, Powell J (eds) (1982) Cancer incidence in five continents. International Agency for Research on Cancer, Lyon, vol 4

144. Seedorf K, Krämmer G, Dürst M, Suhai S, Röwekamp WG (1985) Human papillomavirus type 16 sequence (submitted for publication)

145. Zur Hausen H (1983) Herpes simplex virus in human genital cancer. Int Rev Exptl Pathol 25:307-326

Vaccine Strategies against the Human Retroviruses Associated with AIDS

Introduction

The acquired immune deficiency syndrome (AIDS) is, in general, a blood-borne disorder which is transmitted by a human retrovirus usually termed HTLV–III but also lymphadenopathy-associated virus (LAV) or combinations of the two designations (HTLV–III/LAV or LAV/HTLV–III)[1]. By 1982, 3 years after the disease was recognised, the Center for Disease Control in Atlanta (USA) officially declared AIDS an epidemic[2]. To date, more than 16 000 cases have been reported and one-half of these have been fatal. Equally important is the overwhelming number of individuals, as many as 2 000 000 in the USA, who have been infected with HTLV–III and remain asymptomatic but can transmit the virus as effectively as their diseased counterparts. A healthy virus carrier state which is, for the most part, unrecognised creates the alarming possibility that there will be no obvious barriers between the infected and uninfected population. As would be expected, both the virus and the disease are steadily finding their way into the general population[3], and, in spite of the acute public awareness of this problem, we are faced with a rapidly spreading infectious agent which requires the development of strict countermeasures. These include improved detection of the virus, prevention of further spread and ultimately its elimination from the population.

In man's history there have been numerous instances where life-threatening infectious diseases have been eradicated by immunisation. Paramount examples are the conquest of virus diseases such as polio and smallpox. However, we continue to face new challenges with viruses which have considerable impact on the quality of life for which development of vaccines has been lagging. These include agents such as hepatitis virus, various members of the herpesvirus family and the human papillomaviruses, which infect populations on a large scale. In some parts of the world, the long-term sequelae of infection by some of these agents include the development of malignant neoplasms[4-7].

This is true also for the various members of the human retrovirus family. HTLV–I infection is directly associated with adult T-cell leukaemia[8]. HTLV–II has been linked with hairy cell leukaemia but the full spectrum of its disease potential is not yet defined[9]. HTLV–I is also associated with B-cell neoplasms, although it is not a direct cause[10]. Hence, a variety of diseases can result from infection with these agents, perhaps as a consequence of their ability to alter T-cell function[11]. The same principle applies to HTLV–III, the primary aetiological agent of the acquired immune deficiency syndrome known as AIDS. Among the spectrum of diseases catalogued under the definition of AIDS one finds Kaposi's sarcoma, B-cell lymphomas in the brain and various carcinomas[2]. In none of these neoplasms is there evidence of direct viral causation, but there is little doubt that viruses are involved indirectly. Hence, the consequences of infection by any of these human retroviruses extend well beyond their acute manifestations of leukaemia and AIDS. In that context a careful follow-up of healthy virus carriers may reveal much that lies beneath the surface.

In attempting to devise vaccine strategies against human retroviruses, one is immediately drawn to the issue of previous experience with their animal counterparts. Fortunately, the available information indicates that vaccination against retroviruses is an achievable goal. However, to temper that optimism, the possibility of developing a vaccine against human retroviruses, notably HTLV–III, depends on overcoming considerable obstacles. The purpose of this discussion is to review both sides of this question and to outline a general course for developing effective preventative measures against HTLV–III and, indirectly, against other human retroviruses.

Retrovirus Antigens which Elicit Immunity to Infection

The viral component responsible for the salient immunobiological features of a retrovirus is its major external glycoprotein (gp) (for review, see Reference 12). First the gp is required for infection and presumably mediates the attachment of the virus to the host cell. It is also the viral component that is more directly involved in the phenomenon of interference, as it relates to viral receptors at the cell surface. Finally, the gp specifies the pattern of neutralisation by antiviral antibodies. Consistent with these properties is its strategic location on the outer envelope of virion[13] (see Fig. 6.1).

Another antigen found on the surface of virion is a hydrophobic transmembrane protein (tmp) which non-covalently anchors the gp to the virion[13]. The tmp can either contain or be devoid of carbohydrate, but in every case the degree of glycosylation is considerably less than in the exterior gp. The tmp can also be a target for neutralisation by antibodies, but this is generally weak unless complement is present[14].

The viral gp and tmp are also present in infected cells, concentrated in the budding virion but present at other sites as well which are more uniformly distributed on the cell surface[15]. As such, the gp represents a cellular target for immune attack[16].

Animals infected with retroviruses usually respond with easily detectable humoral immunity against the exterior gp. For the most part these are selective

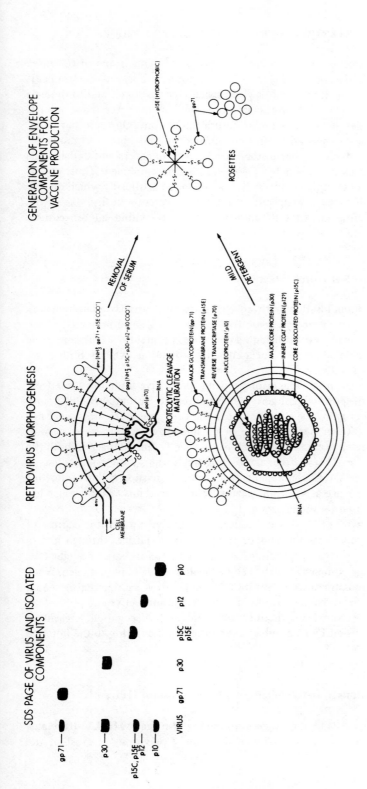

Fig. 6.1 Morphogenesis, structure and composition of a typical murine leukaemia retrovirus. The surface components gp71 (gp) and p15E (tmp) derived from the *env* gene of the virus can be recovered in homogeneous form either as multimers (rosettes) or monomers as a result of shedding from the cell surface[22] or treatment with mild non-ionic detergents[51]

for the infecting agent — i.e. they are *type specific*[17]. This is one of the three immunogenic domains of the external gp. The others represent determinants which are common to all viruses of a given species (*group*) or extend to those in widely different species (*interspecies*)[12]. It is only in rare cases that animals respond to these latter domains under natural conditions. On the other hand, one can immunise animals with virus of purified gp and obtain antibody responses which are much broader in their reactivity than natural antibodies. This is particularly the case when heterologous species are employed. Thus, potent neutralising as well as cytotoxic antibodies can be raised artificially which display strong *group*- and *interspecies*-specific reactivity[12]. Parenthetically, one of the most conserved antigenic sites of antigenic reactivity within all retroviruses resides in the *tmp*[18].

Vaccination against Retrovirus Infections

As noted above, immunisation with gp elicits strong neutralising antibodies as well as antibodies which are cytotoxic for infected cells. Mice immunised with purified gp can, indeed, resist substantial challenges of infectious leukaemogenic virus[19]. The immune response associated with protection exhibits both *type*- and *group*-specific reactivity[19,20].

While monomeric gp is capable of inducing protective immunity, relatively large quantities of purified antigen were required to accomplish this reproducibly[19]. In other animal systems, notably the cat, similar attempts were not successful. On the other hand, the use of gp linked to the tmp so as to form multimeric aggregates resulted in a much more effective immunogen in both the mouse[20] and the cat[21] (see Fig. 6.1). It is likely that a similar principle is involved in the use of viral components from cell culture supernatants following serum starvation for use as a vaccine against feline leukaemia virus[22] which has recently been licensed for use in cats.

Recently, the work of Morein and colleagues[23] has shown that the capture of virus envelope components (gp and tmp) by glycoside lattices through hydrophobic interaction with tmp generates a multimeric matrix structure (ISCOM; immune stimulating complex) which is an unusually powerful immunogen. When compared with monomeric gp, an ISCOM preparation containing an equal amount of gp elicits at least a tenfold increase in the protective end point[24]. It may be that these complex structures are more easily recognised, presented, taken up and processed by macrophages for antigen presentation to the immune system.

Special Considerations in Development of a Vaccine against HTLV-III

A major challenge in developing a successful immunogen against HTLV-III relates to the problem of genomic diversity in this family of viruses[25]. Most of the variability occurs in the exterior glycoprotein portion of the envelope gene[25,26]. The significance of the extensive variability in certain regions of the gp120 is not apparent in relation to the antiviral immune responses occurring in patients. In other words, there is no evidence of a hypervariable immune response which mirrors the genomic changes. However, the presence or absence of humoral anti-viral immunity has not correlated with the presence of infection or the develop-ment of AIDS[27], and the significance of its role remains obscure.

This question has been studied in much greater detail in the lentivirus sub-family of retroviruses, certain members of which share several features with HTLV-III. One such virus, the equine infectious anaemia virus (EIAV), escapes humoral immunity in a unique fashion[28]. The initial infection is met by a vigorous neutralising antibody response, but variants are apparently generated which are refractory to its effect. As the variant replicates, a second round of antibody is produced which is specific for the new virus; but again new variants emerge. By repeating this cycle of neutralisation, mutation and escape, the virus is able to complete its pathogenic mission. Antigenic variation and escape from neutralising antibody also occur with Visna virus[29], whose genomic structure and pathobiology in the infected animal are similar to those of HTLV-III[30,31].

Returning to the issue of HTLV-III, a second major concern relates to the mode of transmission of the virus. More specifically, does the infectious material consist of free virus, virus-infected cells or both? It is likely that each is possible and that none are mutually exclusive. A corollary to this situation is how the virus spreads within the host following the initial infection: again, is it as free virus or via cell-to-cell contact? The probability that both mechanisms are involved is reasonably high. With these considerations in mind, a successful vaccine against HTLV-III infection would have to be capable of eliciting both neutralising antibodies and an immune response that could destroy infected cells. While the presence of virus-specific cellular immunity has been weak or absent[20], antibodies which are cytolytic in the presence of complement or mediate antibody-dependent cellular cytotoxicity (ADCC) have been documented in animal models (for review, see Reference 32). In so far as cell-mediated immunity is concerned, the possible role of viral components other than those associated with the envelope, needs to be considered, as demonstrated recently in other virus systems[32a,32b].

A third issue to consider is the extensive layer of carbohydrate which covers the HTLV-III exterior gp. There are 32 potential glycosylation sites on the molecule such that as much as 40% of its apparent molecular weight on SDS gels, 120 000 daltons (gp120)[33,34], consists of polysaccharide side-chains[35]. This raises the important question of whether the sugar umbrella impedes vaccine development by masking epitopes on the protein backbone which would other-wise be targets for neutralisation. A corollary is whether deglycosylated forms of the gp might be better or at least equally effective immunogens. This possibility has indeed been suggested by the studies of Elder et al.[36]. This is consistent with a number of studies with animal retroviruses showing that the targets for neutral-isation reside on the protein backbone[37]. This is not to say that glycosylation is not important. Clearly, some glycosylation is critical for the appropriate folding of the protein, especially for epitopes consisting of non-contiguous regions, as have been described in studies with the GIX gp of murine retroviruses[38].

Approaches for a Vaccine against HTLV–III

Apart from the question of what constitutes an effective human vaccine are the issues of safety, homogeneity, quantity and economy. Such considerations lead one immediately towards molecular engineering approaches as a first step. This is not unlike the current strategies for developing vaccines against hepatitis B or herpesviruses[39-41]. One must first decide whether to develop recombinant products in bacteria, yeast or mammalian cells for HTLV–III vaccine material. This will depend on the role which carbohydrate plays in the immunogenicity of the gp and the form of the molecule which displays the neutralisation epitopes which are conserved among the sub-strains[26]. If the quantity or quality of common epitopes proves to be a problem, one might be faced with the difficult task of choosing a cocktail of immunogens derived from representative strains.

If linear epitopes can be demonstrated which are effective targets for neutralisation, the possibility of synthetic peptides comes immediately to mind. However, on the basis of current experience with synthetic peptides as immunogens, it is likely that special modes of presentation will be necessary in order to generate protective immune responses against live virus challenges[42]. As indicated above for the native gp, one may wish to consider the ISCOM approach for both the peptide and recombinant materials.

Another attractive method would be to use infectious recombinant viruses. Typically a non-essential region of vaccinia virus, a classical vaccine virus with a known safety record, would be used as the locus for the desired gene, which would then be expressed under the control of vaccinia promoters. The resulting construct would consist of autonomously replicating vaccinia virus which would also express large amounts of properly processed inserted antigen[43,44]. An attractive feature would be that a number of related gp regions could be introduced in sequence, as has been recently demonstrated[45]. Since there are a number of considerations which might mitigate against using vaccinia as a vector (i.e. prior immunisation of the population, possible pathogenicity in certain individuals), non-pathogenic strains of herpesviruses or adenoviruses may also be considered.

A final possibility is the use of anti-idiotypes as immunogens. An anti-idiotype represents the internal image of the relevant epitope within the antigen-combining regions of the antibody. In several experimental systems a proper combination of native antigen and an anti-idiotype to the neutralising antibody induces a powerful and long-lasting protective response within several compartments of the immune system[46].

Animal Models for Testing Efficacy of HTLV–III Vaccines

At the present time there are at least three possibilities for testing the various vaccine possibilities outlined above.

The first derives from studies which demonstrate that chimpanzees can be successfully infected with HTLV–III[47]. These animals sero-convert and become viraemic within 2 months of infection. They also exhibit a transient lymphadenopathy and other immune abnormalities. One could thus directly evaluate the capability of vaccine preparations to block infection by HTLV–III.

One potential drawback of the chimpanzee model is the shortage of animals and appropriate containment facilities to conduct the challenge trials. For this reason attempts are being made to infect with HTLV–III smaller primates such as rhesus monkeys. To date, variable degrees of success have been recorded but none approaches the efficiency of infecting chimpanzees. It appears that prior adaptation of the virus in the rhesus monkey may be necessary to obtain higher infectivity.

In addition to infectivity models, a disease model for AIDS in sub-human primates is mediated by the simian counterpart of STLV–III[48]. This is particularly attractive, since HTLV–III and STLV–III share substantial antigenic cross-reactivity in their envelope glycoproteins[49]. The possibility that cross-protection could occur between these agents should be examined — particularly with regard to the HTLV–III sub-unit vaccines being tested.

Regardless of which model is being used for testing, the issues of genomic diversity and mode of transmission will have to be seriously considered. Hence, the model must be amenable to challenge with different sub-strains of HTLV–III, including those which exhibit the greatest degree of diversity. In addition, the route of inoculation, the challenge dose and the inclusion of infected cells in the challenge will have to be addressed.

Conclusions

Though difficult, the problems associated with devising a successful vaccine against HTLV–III are not insurmountable. The heterogeneity among the virus isolates is balanced by conserved regions which are potential targets for immune attack. While natural antibodies against retroviruses are extremely narrow in their specificity, antibodies raised artificially are much more broadly reactive. Presumably the same situation is operative with HTLV–III and vaccine strategies must focus on the conserved regions. In that context the mode of antigen presentation will be critical to achieve the desired response.

In the same vein the elicitation of immune responses which are effective in dealing with virus-infected cells is an attainable goal. Both cytotoxic and cytophilic antibodies can be obtained in response to immunisation with retroviruses and, as noted earlier, these are extremely active in clearing infected cells in model systems (for review, see Reference 32).

An additional issue which has not been covered in this chapter is that of the role of secretory immunity. Most viruses which are pathogenic in man enter through mucous membranes. There is substantial evidence that secretory immunity is an effective barrier during the early stages of viral infection[50]. In the case of HTLV-III, there is a strong possibility that epithelial surfaces are involved in virus transmission — particularly where the sexual route is concerned. Indeed, there is evidence for the presence of a secretory immune response to HTLV-III when one examines saliva of infected individuals (M. Essex, personal communication). The role of secretory IgA as a line of defence against HTLV-III infection needs to be explored.

It is therefore reasonable, considering the rapidly accumulating knowledge of the structure of HTLV-III structural components coupled with access to modern biotechnology, to be optimistic about development of effective vaccines against HTLV-III disease. If one draws on past experience in animal models, vaccination against retroviruses can guarantee long-term protection against infection and disease. These principles will certainly be applicable to other human diseases associated with retroviruses. Where these are associated with malignant neoplasms, there is a remarkable opportunity to control a cancer by direct attack on the aetiological agent.

References

1. Broder S, Gallo RC (1984) A pathogenic retrovirus (HTLV-III) linked to AIDS. New England Journal of Medicine 311:1292-1297
2. Curran JW, Morgan WM, Hardy AM, Jafe HW, Darrow WW, Dowdle WR (1985) The epidemiology of AIDS: current status and future prospects. Science 229:1352-1357
3. Wong-Staal F, Gallo RC (1985) Human T-lymphotropic retroviruses. Nature 317: 395-403
4. Blumberg BS, London WT (1985) Hepatitis B virus and the prevention of primary cancer of the liver. Journal of the National Cancer Institute 71:267-273
5. Epstein MA, Achong BG (1979) In: Epstein MA, Achong BG (eds) The Epstein-Barr virus. Springer, Berlin, Heidelberg, New York
6. Rapp F, Howett MK (1983) Involvement of herpes simplex virus in cervical carcinoma. In: Chandra P (ed) Biochemical and biological markers of neoplastic transformation. Plenum, New York, 555-572
7. zur Hausen H, Gissmann L, de Villiers EM (1983) Papillomaviruses. In: Chandra P (ed) Biochemical and biological markers of neoplastic transformation. Plenum, New York, p 595-602
8. Poiesz BJ, Ruscetti FW, Gazdar AF, Bunn PA, Minna JD, Gallo RC (1980) Detection and isolation of type C retrovirus particles from fresh and cultured lymphocytes of a patient with cutaneous T-cell lymphoma. Proceedings of the National Academy of Sciences USA 77:7415-7419
9. Kalyanaraman VS, Sarngadharan MG, Robert-Guroff M, Blaynay D, Golde F, Gallo RC (1982) Natural antibodies to human retrovirus HTLV in a cluster of Japanese patients with adult T-cell leukemia. Science 215:975-978
10. Clark J, Saxinger C, Gibbs WN, Lofters W, Lagranade L, Deceulaer K, Ensroth A, Robert-Guroff M, Gallo RC, Blattner W (1985) Seroepidemilogic studies of human T cell leukemia/lymphoma virus type I in Jamaica. International Journal of Cancer 36:37-41

11. Popovic M, Flomenberg N, Volkman DJ, Mann D, Fauci AS, Du Pont B, Gallo RC (1984) Alteration of T-cell function by infection with HTLV-I or HTLV-II. Science 226: 459–462

12. Schafer W, Bolognesi DP (1977) Mammalian C type oncornaviruses: relationship between viral structural and cell surface antigens and their possible significance in immunological defense mechanisms. Contemporary Topics in Immunobiology 6:127–167

13. Bolognesi DP, Montelaro RC, Frank H (1978) Assembly of type C oncornaviruses: a model. Science 199:183–186

14. Fischinger PJ, Schafer W, Bolognesi DP (1976) Neutralisation of homologous and heterologous oncornaviruses by antisera against the p15(E) and gp71 polypeptides of Friend murine leukemia virus. Virology 71:169–184

15. Schwarz H, Hunsmann G, Moennig V, Schafer W (1976) Properties of mouse leukemia viruses. XII. Immunoelectron microscopic studies on viral structural antigens on the cell surface. Virology 69:169–178

16. Hunsmann G, Claviez M, Moennig V, Schwarz H, Schafer W (1976) Properties of mouse leukemia viruses. X. Occurrence of viral structural antigens on the cell surface as revealed by a cytotoxicity test. Virology 69: 157–168

17. Ihle JN, Lee JC, Hanna MG Jr (1976) Characterization of natural antibodies in mice to endogenous leukaemia virus. In: Yuhan JM, Tennant RW, Regan JD (eds) The biology of radiation carcinogenesis. Raven Press, New York, p 261–273

18. Thiel HJ, Broughton EM, Matthews TJ, Schafer W, Bolognesi DP (1981) Interspecies reactivity of type C and D retroviruses p15E and p15C proteins. Virology 111: 270–274

19. Hunsmann G, Moennig V, Schafer W (1975) Properties of mouse leukemia viruses. IX. Active and passive immunization of mice against Friend leukemia with isolated viral GP71 glycoprotein and its corresponding antiserum. Virology 66:327–329

20. Hunsmann G, Schneider J, and Schulz A (1981) Immunoprevention of Friend virus-induced erythroleukemia by vaccination with viral envelope glycoprotein complexes. Virology 113:602–612

21. Hunsmann G, Pedersen NC, Theilen GH, Bayer H (1983) Active immunization with feline leukemia virus envelope glycoprotein suppresses growth of virus-induced feline sarcoma. Immunology 171:233–241

22. Lewis MG, Mathes LE, Olson RG (1981) Protection against feline leukaemia by vaccination with a subunit vaccine. Infection and Immunity 34:888–894

23. Morein B, Sundquist B, Hoglund S, Dalsgaard K, Osterhaus S (1984) Iscom a novel structure for antigenic presentation of membrane proteins from envelope viruses. Nature 308: 457–462

24. Osterhaus A, Weijer K, Uytdehaag F, Jarrett O, Sundquist B, Morein BJ (1985) Induction of protective immune response in cats by vaccination with feline leukemia virus iscom. Journal of Immunology 135:591–596

25. Hahn BH, Gonda MA, Shaw GM, Popovic M, Hoxie JA, Gallo RC, Wong-Staal F (1985) Genomic diversity of the acquired immune deficiency syndrome virus HTLV-III: Different viruses exhibit greatest divergence in their envelope genes. Proceedings of the National Academy of Sciences USA 82:4813–4817

26. Starcich BR, Hahn BH, Shaw GM, et al. (1986) Identification and characterization of conserved and divergent regions in the envelope genes of HTLV-III/LAV, the retrovirus of AIDS. Cell (in preparation)

27. Robert-Guroff M, Brown M, Gallo RC (1985) HTLV-III-neutralizing antibodies in patients with AIDS and AIDS-related complex. Nature 316:72–74

28. Kono Y, Kobayasi K, Fukunaga Y (1973) Antigenic drift of equine infectious anaemia virus in chronically infected horses. Archiv Gesamte Virusforschung 41:1–10

29. Scott JV, Stowring L, Haase AT (1979) Antigenic variation in visna virus. Cell 18: 321–327

30. Gonda MA, Wong-Staal F, Gallo RC, Clements JW, Marayan O, Gilden RV (1985) Sequence of homologous and morphologic similarity of HTLV-III and visna virus, a pathogenic lentivirus. Science 227: 173–177

31. Sonigo P, Alizon M, Staskus K, Dlatzman D, Cole S, Danos O, Retzel E, Tiollais P,

Haase A, Wain-Hobson S (1985) Nucleotide sequence of the visna lentivirus: Relationships to the AIDS virus. Cell 42:369–382

32. Iglehart JD, Weinhold KJ, Ward EC, Matthews TJ, Langlois AJ, Schafer W, Bolognesi DP (1983) Prospects for the immunological management of lethal tumors. Cancer Investigation 1: 409–421

32.a Yewdell JW, Bennink JR, Smith GL, Moss B (1985) Influenza A virus nucleoprotein is a major target antigen for cross-reactive anti-influenza A virus cytotoxic T lymphocytes. Proceedings of the National Academy of Sciences USA 82:178–1789

32.b Townsend ARM, Gotch FM, Davey J (1985) Cytotoxic T cells recognize fragments of the influenza nucleoprotein. Cell 42: 457–467

33. Kitchen LW, Bann F, Sullivan JL, McLane MF, Brettler DB, Levince PH, Essex M (1984) Aetiology of AIDS – antibodies to human T-cell leukaemia virus (type III) in haemophiliacs. Nature 312:367

34. Robey WG, Safai B, Oroszlan S, Arthur LO, Gonda MA, Gallo RC, Fischinger PJ (1985) Characterization of envelope and core structural gene products of HTLV-III with sera from AIDS patients. Science 228:593–595

35. Ratner L, Haseltine W, Patarca R, Livak KJ, Starcich B, Josephs SF, Doran ER, Rafaliski JA, Whitehorn EA, Baumeister K, Ivanoff L, Petteway SR Jr, Pearson ML, Lautenberger JA, Papas TS, Ghrayeb J, Chang NT, Gallo RC, Wong-Staal F (1985) Complete nucleotide sequence of the AIDS virus HTL-III. Nature 313:277–284

36. Elder JH, McGee JS, Alexander S (1985) Carbohydrate side chains of Rauscher leukaemia virus envelope glycoproteins are not required to elicit a neutralizing antibody response. Journal of Virology 57:340–342

37. Schafer W, Fischinger PJ, Collins JJ, Bolognesi DP (1977) Role of carbohydrate in biological functions of Friend murine leukaemia virus gp71. Journal of Virology 22:35–40

38. Pierotti M, DeLeo AB, Pinter A, et al. (1981) The GIX antigen of murine leukemia virus: an analysis with monoclonal antibodies. Virology 112:450

39. Valenzuela P, Coit D, Kuo CH (1985) Synthesis and assembly in yeast of hepatitis B surface antigen particles containing the polyalbumin receptor. Biotechnology 3: 317–320

40. Valenzuela P, Coit D, Medina-Selby MA, Kuo CH, VanNest G, Burke RL, Bull P, Urdea MS, Graves PV (1985) Antigen engineering in yeast: Synthesis and assembly of hybrid hepatitis B surface antigen–herpes simplex 1 gD particles. Biotechnology 3:323–326

41. Berman PW, Gregory T, Crase D, Lasky LA (1985) Protection from genital herpes simplex Type 2 infection by vaccination with Type 1 glycoprotein D. Science 227: 1490–1492

42. Tainer JA, Getzoff ED, Alexander H, Houghton RA, Olson AJ, Lerner RA (1984) The reactivity of anti-peptide antibodies is a function of the atomic mobility of sites in a protein. Nature 312:127–134

43. Paoletti E, Lipinskas BR, Samsonoff C, Mercer S, Panicali D (1984) Construction of live vaccines using genetically engineered poxviruses. Biological activity of vaccinia virus recombinants expressing the hepatitis B virus surface antigen and the herpes simplex virus glycoprotein D. Proceedings of the National Academy of Sciences USA 81:193–197

44. Mackett M, Smith GL, Moss B (1982) Vaccinia virus – a selectable eukaryotic cloning and expression vector. Proceedings of the National Academy of Sciences USA 79:7415–7419

45. Perkus ME, Piccini A, Lipinskas BR, Paoletti E (1985) Recombinant vaccinia virus: immunization against multiple pathogens. Science 229:981–984

46. McNamara M, Gleason K, Kohler H (1984) T-cell helper circuits. Immunological Review 79:87–102

47. Alter HJ, Eichberg JW, Masur H, Saxinger WC, Gallo R, Macher AM, Lane HC, Fauci AS (1984) Transmission of HTLV-III infection from human plasma to chimpanzees: an animal model for AIDS. Science 226:549–552

48. Daniel MD, Letvin NL, King NW, Kannagi M, Sehgal PK, Hunt RD, Kanki PJ, Essex M, Desrosiers RC (1985) Isolation of T-cell tropic HTLV-III-like retroviruses from macaques. Science 228:1201–1204

49. Kanki PJ, McLane MF, King NW Jr, Letvin NL, Hunt RD, Sehgal P, Daniel MD, Desrosiers RC (1985) Serologic identification and characterization of a macaque T-lymphotropic retrovirus closely related to HTLV–III. Science 228: 1199–1201
50. Chanock RM (1971) In: Dayton DH, Small PA, Chanock RM, Kaufman HE, Tomasi TB (eds) The secretory immunologic system. US Government Printing Office, Washington DC
51. Bolognesi DP, Bauer H, Gelderblom H, Huper G (1972) Polypeptides of avian RNA tumor viruses. IV. Components of the viral envelope. Virology 47:551–556

The Role of Cytomegalovirus in Kaposi's Sarcoma and Acquired Immune Deficiency Syndrome

Introduction

Cytomegalovirus (CMV) has been associated with a wide spectrum of clinical syndromes ranging from asymptomatic infections, congenital inclusion disease, mental retardation, infectious mononucleosis-like syndrome, interstitial pneumonia in organ transplants or immunocompromised patients to certain malignancies, particularly Kaposi's sarcoma (KS); the last whether in its classical, endemic or epidemic form[1-3]. The concept that common ubiquitous viruses may be responsible for or have a specific function in the initiation of certain types of human malignancies in individuals with underlying immunodeficiencies appears to be valid for at least two herpesviruses, the Epstein–Barr virus (EBV) and CMV, associated with Burkitt's lymphoma/nasopharyngeal carcinoma and Kaposi's sarcoma, respectively[5-6].

This chapter will focus on CMV and its association with this otherwise rare skin tumour, the latter, surprisingly enough, appearing in an epidemic form since the early 1980s in association with acquired immune deficiency syndrome (AIDS)[7]. We shall summarise the data linking various types of KS with CMV and review the aetiopathogenic mechanisms giving rise to this tumour.

Biological Properties of CMV

The most distinctive biological characteristic of CMV, a member of the herpesvirus sub-family 'beta herpesviridae', is high species specificity. In vitro CMV replicates preferentially in human skin fibroblasts, while in vivo its presence has been identified in a broad spectrum of cells whether derived from the endo-, ecto- or mesoderm[6,8]. It is of interest to note in this context that CMV replication can occur also in endothelial cells[8], which have been identified as the cell of origin of KS[9-11]. Endothelial cells represent a cell type whose actual function regarding the expression of histocompatibility gene(s), particularly of the HLA-DR locus, and their importance in the control of immune responsiveness to viral infections, are still poorly understood. Like other herpesviruses, CMV has the ability to establish persistent infection, to undergo a latent stage and to become reactivated[6]. In fact, long-term latent infection with subsequent recurrence due to allogeneic stimulation or in the immunocompromised host are the most frequent observations recorded, whether in experimental systems of mice or in humans, such as organ transplant patients, promiscuous homosexual men, as well as populations of equatorial African regions, in which diseases due to microbial infections occur frequently, to name malaria as only one example[12-16].

It has been demonstrated[17] that CMV infections increase susceptibility to opportunistic infections and cause a variety of immunological abnormalities[18,19]. The major abnormalities induced during symptomatic infections in renal transplant recipients and during acute mononucleosis-like syndrome appear to be in T-cell function and involve depression of proliferative and cytotoxic responses, as well as gamma-interferon production. Acute infection is associated with reversal of the normal ratio between T4 and T8 cells, reflecting a large absolute increase in T8 cells and a smaller decrease in T4 cells in the peripheral blood. These changes are reminiscent of acute infections with EBV, although T-sub-set aberrations in CMV infections may persist for longer periods (7–12 months)[20,21]. In addition, autoreactive antibodies have been associated with CMV infection as well as the appearance of circulating immune complexes[22,23]. B-lymphocyte responses in vitro appear to show no marked abnormalities[18]. Polymorphonuclear leucocytes are the principal site of virus carriage but it is not known whether this is due to their phagocytic function or is because CMV replicates in granulocyte precursors. Garrett[24] reported that T-cell-enriched populations from 18 renal transplant recipients harboured CMV, whereas B lymphocytes did not.

Investigations to determine the ability of CMV to infect peripheral blood leucocytes in vitro revealed that the virus could infect T and B cells, natural killer cells and monocytes[25]. The infection was abortive, with synthesis of only immediate-early virus-induced polypeptides, including the major 72K protein. Furthermore, infected lymphocytes lost their function of proliferative responses when stimulated with phytohaemagglutinin (PHA). However, if lymphocytes were first stimulated with PHA and then infected, T cells became permissive for productive CMV infection[26]. The increased susceptibility appears to be due to the replication of T cells, since experiments with cell lines established with PHA and T-cell growth factor (TCGF) confirmed this finding. Moreover, when T cells from patients with AIDS, AIDS-related complex (ARC) or asymptomatic homosexual men were analysed, T4 cells appeared to be the predominant subpopulation associated with CMV[27]. Intensive studies have recently succeeded in identifying, isolating and characterising human T-cell-tropic, cytopathic retroviruses, referred to as lymphadenopathy-associated virus (LAV)[28], human T-cell lymphotropic virus, type III (HTLV–III)[29] or AIDS-associated retrovirus (ARV)[30]. They are aetiologically associated with AIDS and have a preferential T4 cell tropism. Since replication of CMV results in cell death, permissiveness of stimulated T cells and, in particular, T4 cells could thus add this virus, in addition to the identified lyric T-cell-tropic retrovirus, to the agents responsible for the great reduction of T4 cells observed in AIDS patients.

That CMV is an oncogenic herpesvirus was first demonstrated in 1973[31]. The identification of the transforming ability of CMV at sub-genomic level was thereafter identified by Nelson et al.[32], using the strain Ad169. They showed that the transforming region is located in a 2.9 kb sub-fragment of the HindIII fragment E with map units between 0.123 and 0.14 on the viral DNA molecule, an area which is heavily transcribed during the immediate-early phase of virus replication. Deletion fragments were constructed from the recombinant plasmid containing the transforming region (pCM4000), and a minimum size sequence for transformation was identified, consisting of only 490 bp[33]. That the CMV genome contains more than one transforming region was identified by a second distinct transforming region in the CMV DNA (Towne strain XbaI fragment E)[34]. It is homologous with the HSV-2 DNA fragment BglII fragment C, known to induce neoplastic transformation of diploid cells. Morphologically, NIH-3T3 cells can be transformed by transfection with these viral DNA fragments and neoplastic growth occurs when they are injected into nude mice.

Association of CMV with Kaposi's Sarcoma

The original reasons why KS deserved investigation as a possible virus-associated malignancy were the following[35,36]: (1) the particular geographic distribution of the tumour; (2) the clinical evolution of the disease; (3) the clinical status as reflected by the histological appearance; (4) the second primary neoplasms frequently found in KS patients; and (5) the multiplicity of lesions. The high incidence and cluster type of occurrence in the indigenous population of equatorial Africa (endemic KS)[37-39] were strongly reminiscent of another virus–cancer association, namely EBV and African Burkitt's lymphoma[4,40]. It is of interest that occurrence in clusters has been also observed in the epidemic form of KS[41,42]. One particular cluster, comprising 40 sexually related homosexual patients with KS and *Pneumocystis carinii* pneumonia, clearly points to the causative role of an infectious agent. In children and young adults in Africa the disease evolves rapidly, and lymphadenopathic involvement is not rare (progressive form)[43,44]. In adults, particularly in the classical form occurring in elderly subjects, the tumour runs a more protracted course and spontaneous regressions can be observed (regressor form). Both types probably reflect differences in immunocompetence, which may also be of crucial importance in the development of the third form of KS, the epidemic type, as well as in renal transplant recipients and other iatrogenically immunosuppressed individuals who develop KS. The histology of the tumour shows a marked lymphomononuclear infiltration compatible with an immunological response to tumour-specific antigens. Second primary neoplasms, which are frequently found in KS patients (particularly lymphomas, mainly Hodgkin's lymphoma), suggest the persistence of a tumour inducer, probably a virus[45]. The multiplicity of lesions in patients with KS suggested to us a multifocal origin compatible with a viral-induced neoplasia.

From 1971 to date, about 250 patients with KS deriving from Zaire, Uganda, Cameroon and Senegal (endemic KS), from Tunisia, France, Italy and the USA (classical KS) and recently from the USA, France and Italy (epidemic KS) have been and/or are being studied in our laboratory. Accumulating serological and molecular epidemiological evidence points to a specific association of CMV in KS of all three forms, as well as probably in kidney transplant recipients and other iatrogenically immunosuppressed patients.

Initially, in order to determine whether there was any evidence of an association of high titres of antibodies to CMV, EBV, HSV-1 or HSV-2 in patients with classical and endemic KS, extensive serological analyses were undertaken. A specific serological association of CMV with classical KS patients, whether from Europe or America, could be demonstrated[46,47]. All patients' sera contained antibodies to CMV, and their geometric mean titres were significantly higher than those in sera from age- and sex-matched melanoma patients as well as in sera from age- and sex-matched healthy blood donors. In contrast, no association was found with EBV, HSV-1 or HSV-2. Patients with endemic KS could not be serologically associated. Ubiquitous viral infections and/or activation of latent viruses occur frequently in subjects living in endemic areas/conditions. As a consequence, a viral association with a specific disease (syndrome) is not easy to establish, since control subjects matched by geographic and socio-epidemiological criteria are equivalently exposed to the agent. The same applies for patients with epidemic KS, as compared with asymptomatic homosexual men

Since endemic KS patients' sera (most of our cases had a progressive form of the disease) failed to demonstrate a serological association, even though nucleic acid sequences homologous to CMV and CMV-determined early antigens were subsequently demonstrated in their tumour biopsy specimens[48,49], we tested one of several possible hypotheses: could low anti-CMV reactivity be due to the formation of antigen-antibody (CMV-Ag-Ab) complexes? This seemed plausible, since we observed during serial antiviral titrations that African patients' sera frequently had anticomplementary activity (Giraldo, unpublished observations). Therefore, sera from equatorial African patients were recently tested for circulating immune complexes (CIC) by the Raji cell radioimmune assay[50]. They were found to have significantly increased levels of CIC by comparison with healthy individuals. When divided into sub-groups based on the clinical stage of disease, a statitistically significant difference was found between progressor and regressor patients. A correlation of CIC levels with stage of disease could be identified: regressors' sera had low CIC, while progressors' sera had high CIC; regressors going to progressor stage passed from low to high CIC (Giraldo et al., in preparation). Furthermore, an inverted correlation was shown in progressors having high levels of CIC but low antibody titres to CMV, while regressors had low levels of

CIC but high antibody titres to CMV. Normal African control subjects were similar to regressors. Preliminary results on sera with high CIC activity using physicochemical procedures similar to those used by Stango et al.[51] have shown that CIC reactive substances were in fact acid-dissociable and contained 7S IgG antibodies. When tested in an anticomplement immunofluorescence (ACIF) test using human fibroblasts infected with CMV for 48 h (CMV late antigens), they were positive, while uninfected fibroblasts were negative. These findings indicate that CMV–Ag–Ab complexes represent an important component of the CIC activity in KS patients with progressive stage of disease and can explain the low serological reactivity to CMV in progressor patients.

In order to strengthen the serological association of CMV with KS, nucleic acid hybridisation studies were undertaken on cellular DNA and RNA from KS biopsy specimens, mainly from endemic but also from one classical KS patient, as well as a search for CMV-determined early antigens in tumour biopsies and early cell cultures derived from them[48,49]. In the first study, using ^{3}H-labelled Towne strain viral DNA, we were able to identify CMV DNA in 3 of 8 endemic KS biopsies. Applying renaturation kinetics, we estimated that as little as 0.1–0.2 viral genome per cell could be detected. Furthermore, we suggested that either as little as 1 molecule of the entire genome was present in 1 of every 5–10 cells or only a single unique fragment of the genome was present in every cell. CMV-determined early antigens were detected in 7 of 31 biopsies and in 4 of 12 KS cell lines with early culture history when tested by ACIF. Boldogh et al.[49], using a ^{32}P-labelled CMV DNA probe from the entire genome of the Towne strain, identified CMV RNA in 5 of 10 KS biopsies. CMV DNA was detected in 3 of 10 tumours analysed. Moreover, it was estimated that 0.05 genome equivalent per cell could be detected. By use of ACIF, CMV-determined antigens were found in 8 of 10 KS biopsies. That CMV RNA and CMV-related antigens are present also in epidemic KS biopsies was subsequently demonstrated by Drew et al.[15] and by Fenoglio et al.[52] There was a concordance observed between immunoperoxidase staining for factor VIII, a feature of endothelial cells, in focally positive neoplastic tissue and a precise localisation of autoradiographic grains (in-situ cytological hybridisation technique for the detection of CMV-specific mRNA) over proliferating KS cells[11]. The identification of nucleic acid sequences homologous to CMV but not to EBV or HSV, as well as the detection of CMV gene products in tumour biopsies and/or early cell cultures derived from them, is an important criterion in establishing the type of virus–cancer association. The detection of CMV early antigens but not late antigens[48,53], and the failure to demonstrate cytomegaly, nuclear inclusions or virus particles in primary biopsies[11,48], rule out a simple passenger role for this virus or a preferential site for virus replication in neoplastic tissue. Furthermore, positive nucleic acid hybridisation results were recently obtained at sub-genomic level in biopsy specimens from classical, endemic and epidemic KS patients, cosmid and plasmid probes containing CMV DNA sequences free of cell DNA homologies being used as hybridising probe[11,54–57].

Kaposi's Sarcoma and Acquired Immune Deficiency Syndrome

The evidence for an association between CMV and KS is summarised in Table 7.1. It would be surprising if CMV did not contribute substantially to the immune defects observed in the various forms of KS. CMV and EBV are the most frequent pathogens in equatorial Africans and in AIDS patients, particularly homosexual men, and viral antibodies are present in high titres in such populations[14-16,46,47,58]. CMV infections induce immunosuppression and cause abnormal T-cell sub-sets[18]. Promiscuous homosexual men have shown a reduced T4/T8 ratio due to a high frequency of sexually transmitted infections[59]. That homosexual men experience multiple episodes of CMV infections was identified by a high prevalence of IgM antibodies and frequent isolation of the virus from semen[14-16]. Therefore, most probably a combined T-cell assault launched by T-cell-tropic retrovirus and CMV, or a combined assault against both T and B cells by T-cell-tropic retroviruses, CMV and EBV, takes place. The use of immuno-suppressive drugs might also compound CMV-induced hyporesponsiveness in patients with AIDS, as well as frequent other microbial infections in equatorial Africans (e.g. holoendemic malaria), immunosuppressive therapy or older age; all these conditions are frequently associated with the various forms of KS[3,5,60].

Table 7.1 Evidence for an association between CMV and Kaposi's sarcoma (classical, endemic and epidemic form)

All patients with KS are CMV seropositive[15,16,46,47,58]

Specific serological association with CMV but not with EBV, HSV-1 or HSV-2[46,47]

Appearance of CIC can be associated with CMV in KS patients' sera (endemic form) (Giraldo et al., in preparation)

CMV antibody titres are inversely correlated with T4 cell concentration (epidemic KS)[58]

Identification of CMV DNA in KS biopsy specimens using complete viral genome DNA as probe[48,49]

Identification of CMV DNA in KS biopsy specimens using subgenomic viral fragment(s) free of cellular DNA as probe[11,54-57]

Identification of CMV RNA in KS biopsy specimens using complete viral genome DNA as probe[15,48,49]

Identification of CMV RNA in KS biopsy specimens using subgenomic viral fragment(s) free of cellular DNA as probe[57]

Identification of CMV early antigens in KS biopsies and early cell cultures derived from them[15,48,49]

CMV can be isolated from urine, semen, liver, lung tissue (epidemic form)[15,16]; on rare occasions from tumour biopsy in tissue culture (lymph node involvement; endemic form)[36]

CMV infections and/or reactivation of endogenous virus are most common and severe in renal transplant patients, who develop KS with high frequency[13,24]

CIC — circulating immune complexes
HSV — herpes simplex virus

Aetiopathogenic Mechanisms Evolving to Kaposi's Sarcoma

A recent retrospective seroepidemiological analysis conducted on a large group of patients with endemic KS from various equatorial African countries, most of them with a progressive type of disease, reminiscent of the epidemic form of KS (bled between 1971 and 1978), revealed that none of them had antibodies to ARV by indirect immunofluorescence test[61], while Western blot analysis on a few questionable sera revealed positivity only against one or two viral polypeptides of LAV (Chermann et al., personal communication). These data suggest to us that a direct involvement of ARV in the development of KS can be excluded and lead us to think that the virus was only sporadically there at that time, possibly in a latent stage — at least in the patients tested by us. However, a *two-step model* for an infectious agent pathogenesis of AIDS/KS (epidemic KS) is a strong possibility. It is highly probable that in a *first step* a combined assault against both T and B cells takes place — particularly by LAV/HTLV-III/ARV in concert with CMV and EBV. The last two viruses are immunosuppressive by themselves and are much more common than other herpesviruses in nearly all patients with AIDS and ARC. The specific involvement of CMV in the induction of KS, or of EBV in Burkitt's lymphoma, as well as herpes simplex virus (HSV) or human papillomavirus (HPV) in squamous cell carcinoma, has to be considered as a *second step*.

Chronic inflammations due to persistent infection(s), often by CMV and EBV, lead frequently to generalised lymphadenopathy. As a consequence, synthesis of angiogenesis factors[62] might be increased, which would result in an activation of endothelial cells. Immunogenetic control (HLA-DR5 versus HLA-DR3) might influence at this point the outcome of the disease. If the patient is HLA-DR5-positive but HLA-DR3-negative, there could be a higher probability that the syndrome progresses to further complications — i.e. KS. The HLA-DR antigen function could be at the level of the immune response genes controlling mainly cell-mediated immunity and/or at the receptor level of activated endothelial cells for CMV infection.

In vitro transformation experiments indicate that the virus is involved in the initiation of transformation, while other factors (cocarcinogens, activation of cellular oncogenes) might be required for the maintenance of the transformed phenotype[63]. As for KS, endothelial cells which are permissive for CMV infection are the prime target for these events, since they are prominent in the constitution of the tumour tissue. How does CMV act in transformation? Does the virus act as a mutagen, and is transformation the result of a 'hit-and-run' mechanism? The failure to detect specific viral nucleic acid sequences or proteins in all KS points in that direction. Moreover, transforming CMV DNA fragment(s) contain sequences similar to the structure of insertion sequence (IS)-like elements[64]. A temporary 'hit-and-run' or a permanent insertion into the cell genome could provide a promoter/insertion type of activation of endogenous viral oncogenes and/or flanking cellular oncogenes. Another possibility could be similar to the finding of HSV-2 and HPV DNA sequences in the same tumour (cervical carcinoma)[65] — namely, CMV and another common virus could interact to provide an initiation/promotion relationship for transformation.

Conclusion

Malignancies occurring with a short latency period in patients undergoing marked immunosuppression can be suspected of being virus-induced, since efficient tumour surveillance is evident only in such a situation. Moreover, a cluster occurrence of disease among close-contact individuals is usually taken as evidence of an infectious nature of the conditions. When a transmissible agent is taken into account, this could mean that with the epidemic of AIDS and KS, KS would be the first transmissible malignancy with a short incubation time discovered in *humans*.

Acknowledgements

This study was supported by a grant from C.N.R. 'Oncologia', the Associazione Italiana per la Ricerca sul Cancro and the Italian Ministry of Health.

References

1. Weller TH (1971) The cytomegaloviruses: Ubiquitous agents with protean clinical manifestations. New England Journal of Medicine 285:203-214
2. Lang DJ (1972) Cytomegalovirus infection in organ transplantation and post-perfusion, an hypothesis. Archiv Gesamte Virusforschung 37:365-377
3. Giraldo G, Beth E (1985) Kaposi's sarcoma today. In: Stone J (ed) Dermatologic immunology and allergy. Mosby, St. Louis, ch 57, p 815-825
4. Epstein MA, Achong BG (1979) The relationship of the Epstein–Barr virus to Burkitt's lymphoma. In: Epstein MA, Achong BG (eds) The Epstein–Barr virus. Springer, Berlin, ch 14, p 321-329
5. Giraldo G, Beth E, Buonaguro FM (1984) Kaposi's sarcoma: a natural model of inter-relationships between viruses, immunologic responses, genetics and oncogenesis. In: Giraldo G, Beth E (eds) Epidemic of acquired immune deficiency syndrome and Kaposi's sarcoma, antibiotics and chemotherapy, 32nd edn. Karger, Basle, p 1-11
6. Rapp F (1984) Cytomegalovirus and carcinogenesis. Journal of National Cancer Institute 72:783-787
7. Center for Disease Control (1981) Kaposi's sarcoma and pneumocystis pneumonia among homosexual men. New York City and California. Morbidity and Mortality Weekly Report 30:305-308
8. Myerson D, Hackman R, Nelson JA, Ward DC, McDougall JK (1983) Widespread presence of histologically occult cytomegalovirus. Human Pathology 15:430-439
9. Guarda LG, Silva EG, Ordanez NG, Smith JL (1981) Factor VIII in Kaposi's sarcoma. American Journal of Clinical Pathology 76:197-200
10. Nadji M, Morales AR, Ziegles-Weissman J, Penneys NS (1981) Kaposi's sarcoma: immunohistologic evidence for an endothelial origin. Archives of Pathology and Laboratory Medicine 105:274-275
11. McDougall JK, Nelson JA, Myerson D, Beckmann AM, Galloway DA (1984) HSV, CMV and HPV in human neoplasia. Journal of Investigative Dermatology 83:72s-76s

12. Olding LB, Jensen FC, Oldstone MBA (1975) Pathogenesis of cytomegalovirus infections. I. Activation of virus from bone marrow-derived lymphocytes by in vitro allogeneic reactivation. Journal of Experimental Medicine 141:561–572

13. Fiala M, Payne JE, Berne TV, Moore TC, Henle W, Montgomerie JZ, Chatterjee SN, Guze LB (1975) Epidemiology of cytomegalovirus infection after transplantation and immunosuppression. Journal of Infectious Diseases 132:421–433

14. Drew WL, Mintz L, Miner RC, Sands M, Ketterer B (1981) Prevalence of CMV infections in homosexual men. Journal of Infectious Diseases 143:188–192

15. Drew WL, Miner RC, Ziegler JL, Gulett JH, Abrams DI, Conant MA, Huang E–S, Groundwater JR, Volberding P, Mintz L (1982) Cytomegalovirus and Kaposi's sarcoma in young homosexual men. Lancet i:125–127

16. Quinnan GV Jr, Mazur H, Rook AH, Armstrong G, Frederick WR, Epstein J, Manischewitz JF, Macher AM, Jackson L, Ames J, Smith HA, Parker M, Pearson GR, Parillo J, Mitchell C, Straus SE (1984) Herpesvirus infections in the acquired immune deficiency syndrome. Journal of the American Medical Association 252:72–77

17. Rand KH, Pollard RB, Merigan TC (1978) Increased pulmonary superinfections in cardiac transplant patients undergoing primary cytomegalovirus infections. New England Journal of Medicine 298:951–953

18. Hirsch MS (1984) Cytomegalovirus-leukocyte interactions. In: Plotkin SA, Michelson S, Pagano JS, Rapp F (eds) CMV: pathogenesis and prevention of human infection, March of Dimes Birth Defects Foundation, 20th edn. Alan R Liss, New York, p 161–173

19. Rytel MW, Aguilar-Torres FG, Baley J, Heim LR (1978) Assessment of the status of cell-mediated immunity in cytomegalovirus-infected renal allograft recipients. Cellular Immunology 37:31–40

20. Reinherz EL, O'Brien C, Rosenthal P, Schlossman SF (1980) The cellular basis for viral induced immunodeficiency: analysis by monoclonal antibodies. Journal of Immunology 125:1269–1274

21. Carney WP, Rubin RH, Hoffman RA, Hansen WP, Healey K, Hirsch MS (1981) Analysis of T cell subsets in cytomegalovirus mononucleosis. Journal of Immunology 126: 2114–2116

22. Kantor GL, Goldbey LS, Johnson BL (1970) Immunologic abnormalities induced by postperfusion cytomegalovirus infection. Annals of Internal Medicine 73:553–558

23. Olding LB, Kingsbury DT, Oldstone MBA (1976) Pathogenesis of cytomegalovirus infection. Distribution of viral products, immune complexes and autoimmunity during latent murine infection. Journal of General Virology 33:267–280

24. Garrett HM (1982) Isolation of human cytomegalovirus from peripheral blood T cells of renal transplant patients. Journal of Laboratory and Clinical Medicine 99:92–97

25. Rice GPA, Oldstone MBA (1984) Nature of the infection of human lymphocytes by cytomegalovirus. In: Proceedings 9th International Herpesvirus Workshop, Seattle. Abstract, p 52

26. St. Jeor SC, Smiley B, Hudig D, Redelman D (1984) Replication of cytomegalovirus in human T lymphocytes. In: Proceedings 9th International Herpesvirus Workshop, Seattle. Abstract, p 133

27. Spector SA, Lavine JE, McCutchan JA, Hirata KK, Neuman TR, Richman DD (1984) Detection of human cytomegalovirus DNA in leukocytes of homosexual men with acquired immunodeficiency syndrome (AIDS). In: Proceedings 9th International Herpesvirus Workshop, Seattle. Abstract, p 94

28. Barré-Sinoussi F, Chermann JC, Rey F, Nugeyre MT, Chamaret S, Gruest J, Dauguet C, Axler-Blin C, Vezinet-Brun F, Rouzioux C, Rozenbaum W, Montagnier L (1983) Isolation of a T-tropic retrovirus from a patient at risk for acquired immune deficiency syndrome (AIDS). Science 220:868–871

29. Gallo RC, Salahuddin SZ, Popovic M, Shearer GM, Kaplan M, Haynes BF, Palker TJ, Redfield R, Oleske J, Safai B, White G, Foster P, Markham PD (1984) Frequent isolation of cytopathic retrovirus (HTLV–III) from patients with AIDS and at risk for AIDS. Science 224:500–503

30. Levy JA, Hoffman AD, Kramer SM, Landis JA, Shimabukuro JM, Oshiro LS (1984)

Isolation of lymphocytopathic retrovirus from San Francisco patients with AIDS. Science 225:840–842

31. Albrecht T, Rapp F (1973) Malignant transformation of hamster embryo fibroblasts following exposure to ultraviolet-irradiated human cytomegalovirus. Virology 55:53–61

32. Nelson JA, Fleckenstein B, Galloway DA, McDougall JK (1982) Transformation of NIH 3T3 cells with cloned fragment of human cytomegalovirus strain Ad169. Journal of Virology 43:83–91

33. Nelson JA, Fleckenstein B, Jahn G, Galloway DA, McDougall JK (1984) Structure of the transforming region of human cytomegalovirus Ad169. Journal of Virology 49: 109–115

34. Clanton DJ, Jariwalla RJ, Kress C, Rosenthal LJ (1983) Neoplastic transformation by a cloned human cytomegalovirus DNA fragment uniquely homologous to one of the transforming regions of herpes simplex virus. Proceedings of the National Academy of Sciences USA 80:3826–3830

35. Giraldo G, Beth E, Coeur P, Vogel CL, Dhru DS (1972) Kaposi's sarcoma: a new model in the search for viruses associated with human malignancies. Journal of the National Cancer Institute 49:1495–1507

36. Giraldo G, Beth E, Haguenau F (1972) Herpes-type particles in tissue culture of Kaposi's sarcoma from different geographic regions. Journal of the National Cancer Institute 49:1509–1526

37. Rogoff MG (1968) Age, sex and tribal incidence in Kenya. Cancer in Africa, East African Medical Journal, p 445–448

38. Templeton AC, Hutt MSR (1973) Distribution of tumours in Africa. In: Templeton AC (ed) Recent results in cancer research. Springer, Berlin, p 1–22

39. McHardy J, Williams EH, Geser A, De-Thé G, Beth E, Giraldo G (1984) Endemic Kaposi's sarcoma: incidence and risk factors in the West Nile district of Uganda. International Journal of Cancer 33:203–212

40. Pike MC, Williams EH, Wright D (1967) Burkitt's lymphoma in the West Nile district of Uganda 1961–65. British Medical Journal 2:395–399

41. Center for Disease Control (1982) A cluster of Kaposi's sarcoma and Pneumocystis carinii pneumonia among homosexual male residents of Los Angeles and Orange Counties, California. Morbidity and Mortality Weekly Report 31:305–307

42. Auerbach DM, Darrow WW, Jaffe HW, Curran (1984) A cluster of cases of the acquired immune deficiency syndrome: patients linked by sexual contact. American Journal of Medicine 76:487–492

43. Taylor JF, Templeton AC, Vogel CL, Ziegler J, Kyalwazi SK (1971) Kaposi's sarcoma in Uganda: a clinico-pathological study. International Journal of Cancer 8:122–135

44. Kyalwazi SK (1981) Kaposi's sarcoma: clinical features, experience in Uganda. In: Schönfeld H, Hahn FE (eds) Antibiotics and chemotherapy, 29th edn. Karger, Basle, p 59–67

45. Safai B, Miké V, Giraldo G, Beth E, Good RA (1980) Association of Kaposi's sarcoma with second primary malignancies: possible etiopathogenic implications. Cancer 45: 1472–1479

46. Giraldo G, Beth E, Kourilsky FM, Henle W, Henle G, Miké V, Huraux JM, Andersen HK, Gharbi MR, Kyalwazi KS, Puissant A (1975) Antibody patterns of herpesivruses in Kaposi's sarcoma: serologic association of European Kaposi's sarcoma with cytomegalovirus. International Journal of Cancer 15:839–848

47. Giraldo G, Beth E, Henle W, Henle G, Miké V, Safai B, Huraux JM, McHardy J, De-Thé G (1978) Antibody pattern to herpesviruses in Kaposi's sarcoma. II. Serologic association for American Kaposi's sarcoma with cytomegalovirus. International Journal of Cancer 22:126–131

48. Giraldo G, Beth E, Huang E-S (1980) Kaposi's sarcoma and its relationship to cytomegalovirus (CMV). III. CMV DNA and CMV-early antigens in Kaposi's sarcoma. International Journal of Cancer 26:23–29

49. Boldogh I, Beth E, Huang E-S, Kyalwazi SK, Giraldo G (1981) Kaposi's sarcoma. IV. Detection of CMV DNA, CMV RNA and CMNA in tumor biopsies. International Journal of Cancer 28:469–474

50. Theofilopoulos AN, Wilson CB, Dixon FJ (1976) The Raji cell radioimmune assay for detecting immune complexes in human sera. Journal of Clinical Investigation 57: 169–182

51. Stagno S, Volanakis JE, Reynolds DW, Stroud R, Alford CA (1977) Immune complexes in congenital and natal cytomegalovirus infections in man. Journal of Clinical Investigation 60:838–845

52. Fenoglio CM, Oster MW, Gerfo PL, Reynolds T, Edelson R, Patterson JAK, Madeiros E, McDougall JK (1982) Kaposi's sarcoma following chemotherapy of testicular carcinoma in homosexual men: demonstration of CMV RNA in sarcoma cells. Human Pathology 13:955–959

53. Civantos F, Penneys NS, Haines G (1982) Kaposi's sarcoma: absence of cytomegalovirus. Journal of Investigative Dermatology 79:79–80

54. Shaw S, Spector D, Abrams D, Gottlieb M (1984) Characterization of HCMV sequences in Kaposi's sarcoma tissues from AIDS patients. In: Plotkin SA, Michelson S, Pagano JS, Rapp F (eds) CMV: pathogenesis and prevention of human infection, March of Dimes Birth Defects Foundation, 20th edn. Alan R Liss, New York, p 476

55. McDougall JK, Buonaguro FM, Galloway DA, Nelson JA, Smith PP (1984) DNA virus and EM studies in AIDS. In: Gottlieb MS, Groopman JE (eds) Acquired immune deficiency syndrome. Alan R Liss, New York, p 139–156

56. Rüger R, Burmester GR, Kalden JR, Fleckenstein B (1984) Search for cytomegalovirus DNA in hematopoietic cells from homosexual men with AIDS or lymphadenopathy, and in Kaposi's sarcoma and other tissues. In: Proceedings 9th International Herpesvirus Workshop, Seattle. Abstract, p 93

57. Harvey J, Downing R, Eglin R, Bayley A (1984) Cytomegalovirus DNA in Kaposi's sarcoma. In: Proceedings 15th Meeting of the European Tumour Virus Group, Urbino. Abstract, p 59

58. Marmor M, Friedman-Kien AE, Zoller-Pazner S, Stahl RE, Rubinstein P, Laubenstein L, Williams DC, Klein RJ, Spigland I (1984) Kaposi's sarcoma in homosexual men: a seroepidemiologic case-control study. Annals of Internal Medicine 100:809–815

59. Kornfield H, Vande Stouwe RA, Lange M, Reddy MM, Grieco MH (1982) T-lymphocyte subpopulations in homosexual men. New England Journal of Medicine 307:729–731

60. Giraldo G, Beth E, Kyalwazi SK (1984) The role of cytomegalovirus in Kaposi's sarcoma. In Williams AO, O'Connor GT, De-Thé GB, Johnson CA (eds) Virus-associated cancers in Africa. IARC Pub no 63, Lyon, France, p 583–606

61. Giraldo G, Beth–Giraldo E, Levy JA, Chermann JC (1985) Prevalence of antibodies to ARV/LAV-1 in African patients with Kaposi's sarcoma prior to the epidemic of AIDS. In: Proceedings International Conference on AIDS, Atlanta. Abstract, p 52

62. Taylor S, Folkman J (1982) Protamine is an inhibitor of angiogenesis. Nature 297: 307–312

63. Huang E-S, Boldogh I, Baskar JF, Mar E-C (1984) The molecular biology of human cytomegalovirus and its relationship to various human cancers. In: Giraldo G, Beth E (eds) The role of viruses in human cancer. Elsevier Science Publishers, Amsterdam, vol 2, 169–194

64. Galloway DA, Nelson JA, McDougall JK (1984) Small fragments of herpesvirus DNA with transforming activity contain insertion sequence-like structures. Proceedings of the National Academy of Sciences USA 81:4736–4740

65. McDougall JK, Smith P, Tamini HK, Tolentino E, Galloway DA (1984) Molecular biology of the relationship between herpes simplex virus-2 and cervical cancer. In: Giralso G, Beth E (eds) The role of viruses in human cancer. Elsevier Science Publishers, Amsterdam, vol 2, p 59–71

Subject Index